Staying Ageless in 50 Ways

Overcoming social and psychological cues

that age us

Vol. 2

Danae and Durand

Preface

This is a set of pieces about ageing, but not about what to expect as the years pass. More specifically it is about how we age in accordance with our expectations about what ageing is – ideas we have picked up from media images, science and friends and relatives. It discusses ways of how *not* to grow old, how *not* to give in to social cues, and how to avoid the slow decline towards mental and physical infirmity. The medical advice on healthy ageing is clear: we can slow down the process by healthy living. But this is not just about healthy living; it is about consciousness itself, the way our thoughts and assumptions affect our cells and organs. There is increasing evidence from the new science of epigenetics that the body reads the mind, not the other way round. So this is about how to stay young, not just at heart but in a way that will lead to you having to lie about your age to avoid the stunned silences. There is a way to defy not only received ideas but Nature herself. This is about changing reality.

Growing old is inevitable, they say. This is about why that assumption is wrong.

Contents

Older Mothers

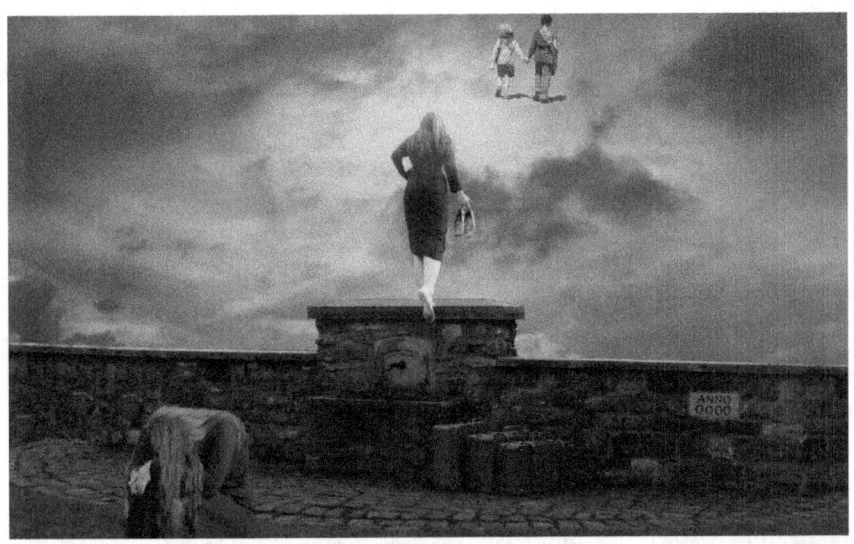

Nature, until now, has been unfair. Men have always been able to continue to reproduce until death, but women's fertility screeches to a halt mid-life.

But despite this it is now quite normal to be a first time mother at forty. The proportion of first births to women 35+ has increased eightfold since 1970. The oldest recorded natural mother gave birth at 59 in the UK in 2007.

As life expectancy continues to increase, women will want to continue to have children into their forties and beyond. Currently most women's eggs have run out by the time they are fifty, and any births after that are almost always either from donor eggs or from ovarian tissue transplant from tissue frozen earlier because of cancer treatment. There have been at the very least raised eyebrows and some virulent condemnations of the few cases of sixty and seventy year old mothers (from donor eggs) who were, according to the critics, unlikely to live long enough to bring up their children. Indeed this was the case of Maria del Carmen Bousada who had twin boys at sixty-six and died two years later of stomach cancer. However, had she lived as long as her mother (101), tongues would not have wagged quite so much.

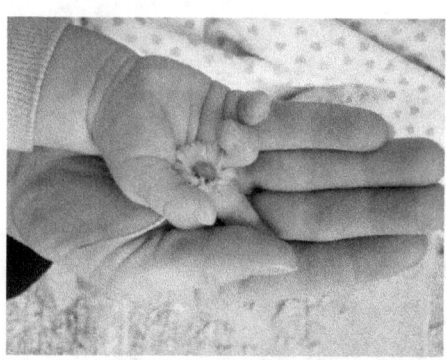

Increased life expectancy can often mean new relationships and the desire to have children with later partners; donor eggs, even if IVF were allowed in all countries at any age (and it's not), are not the solution for most women, especially those with biological children already. Artificial techniques such as freezing eggs and embryos have not been proven to be safe because of the possible damage done by the formation of ice crystals. As research into adult stem cells continues perhaps there will soon be a way to create new eggs from any cell.

Despite the fact more people are living longer, the age of menopause has not changed. Reversing the menopause has been shown to be possible with human growth hormone, but as yet it is not known whether mindfulness techniques and combating social conditioning has any effect on the age of menopause. The word certainly produces anxiety in women, since they fear it signifies the end of their sexual desirability – delaying menopause would therefore mean the ability to continue to look young and fresh for longer. A team led by biologist Rama Singh at McMaster's Dept. of biology has concluded menopause only occurs because men select younger women, rendering menstruation pointless in older women. It is true that few other species manifest menopause, and the prevailing theory until now has been that menopause occurs to allow grandmothers to help their daughters rear more children in quick succession. However, Singh disagrees, claiming that, "If there were no preference against older women, we would be reproducing like men throughout life." Men therefore are to blame for the menopause she claims. If women had historically been the ones to select younger mates, the situation would have been reversed, with men losing fertility. Longevity is not inherited by gender, so women continue to live past their fertility because men remain fertile – and therefore useful to Nature – throughout their lives.

Without the spectre of the menopause, women could finally relax about finding a partner quickly. It would be hugely beneficial for human relationships (many of us are fifty before we understand what the hell's been going on). The pressure would be off, and personal issues and decisions about who we really want to have children with and whether we want them at all could be worked through without the horrible sound of the biological clock ticking away. Epigenetic changes due to lifestyle would have more time to benefit later generations. Big differences in age between siblings and family members who only share one parent might seem irresponsible, but the nuclear family is a recent phenomenon. In the 19th century, when average life expectancy was less than fifty, remarriage was common. Imagine a world where women would no longer have to fear breaking a bone due to osteoporosis, or where the career/motherhood dilemma was finally resolved.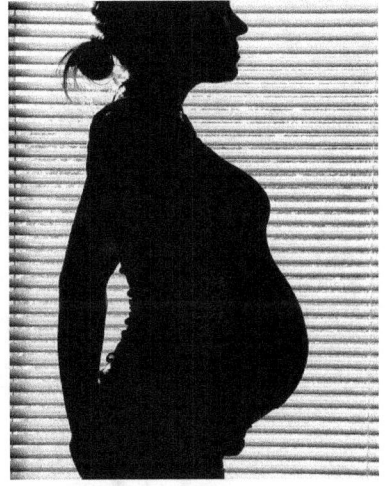

The hive mind objection to anyone looking to extend youth – that it is cheating Nature, that it is weird and selfish – is never voiced more loudly than when it comes to reproduction. However, wisdom and maturity often produce better mothers, and those practising life extension may have spiritual and health perspectives that can only be beneficial to their children. Moreover, the onset of health problems that can accompany the menopause means it is in the interests of society to investigate whether it is time to explore ways of combating this old trick of Nature. If people are remaining healthier for longer older parents will no longer suffer from the disadvantage of being less energetic. Seventy year old mothers may sound grisly to most, but in a world where life will soon be extended to 120, or even 150 for more than the odd outlier, it will perhaps not be quite so peculiar. If the fifty year olds of today are like the thirty year olds of yesteryear, there is nothing to say the seventy and eighty year olds of tomorrow – those who practice staying ageless – will be like the forty year olds of today. Some already are.

Photo Credit: mahalie via Compfight cc
Photo Credit: h.koppdelaney via Compfight cc

Difficult People

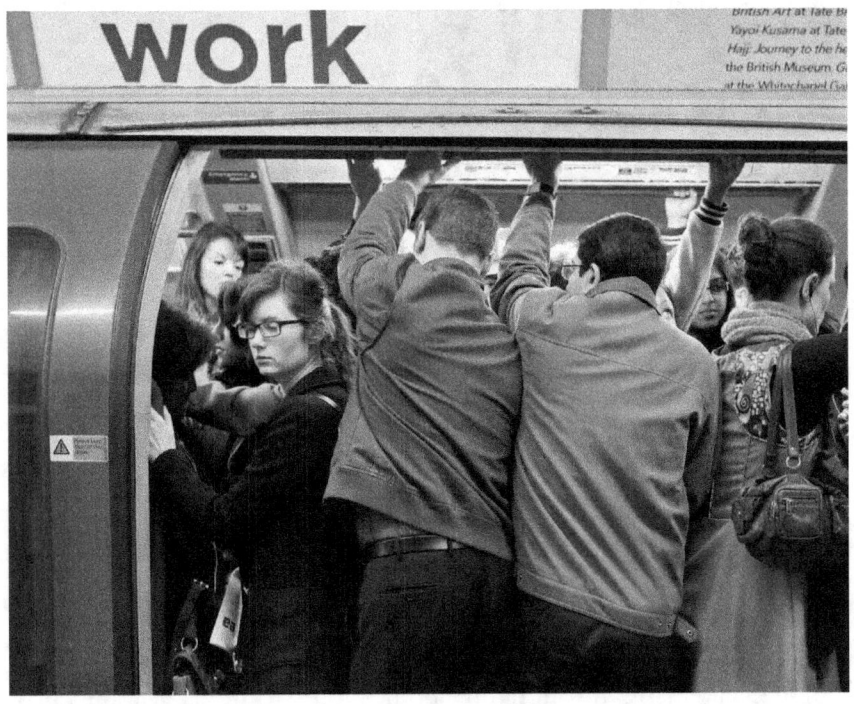

There are 6.4 billion people out there and conflict is a fact of life. Of those 6.4 billion, obsessive compulsives make up 8%, paranoids 4%, schizophrenics 3%, 2% are borderline personality disordered, 5% are chronically depressed and 1% are psychopaths. And those are just the most common disorders. Chances are that even if the only thing we do every day is pop out to buy a loaf of bread, sooner or later one of these people is going to cross our path. This post assumes we are not the difficult person. It assumes we are used to serious soul searching and have not caused conflict through thoughtlessness or aggressive or irresponsible behaviour.

Well....anyone left still listening?

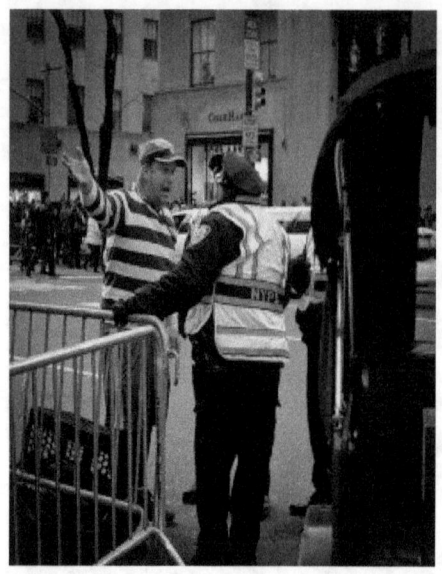

But seriously, although we all overreact sometimes, have our buttons pushed, have impatient days, get angry with slow or foolish individuals etc., there is no doubt that there are also a whole lot of personality disordered people out there living "normal" lives with whom we come into regular contact and whose aggressive, unreasonable and sometimes downright weird behaviour knocks us off our guard.

Some of them are in our own families, some are at work, some pop out of nowhere when we were minding our own business…many are very difficult to avoid.

So….when these people do crazy things, how can we stop our stress levels rocketing, our blood pressure soaring and untold DNA damage careering through our bodies preparing us for an early grave?

The dilemma is this: if we are completely Zen, withdraw, stay silent, do not voice our discontent, although further external conflict may be avoided it is possible we are setting ourselves up for a long period of internal conflict while we deal with feelings of injustice, resentment and frustration. And let us make no mistake….turning over what we might have said, what we should have done and eating ourselves away inside with feelings of outrage at what has been done to us is just as bad….correction, is worse for our health than screaming back at the lunatic who caused this situation in the first place.

However, silence is often far more powerful than throwing a tantrum. So how on earth can we live peaceful, mindful, stress-free lives in a world like ours?

Here are just a few examples of possible reactions to difficult people:

Family members and friends :

Here we mean a family member or friend who fails to respect our boundaries – basically this means treating us as less important than them or even as a non-person. Example : a parent who openly favours another sibling, a family member or flatmate who never knocks before entering our room or who uses our stuff without asking, a relative who never acknowledges we may have feelings or needs.

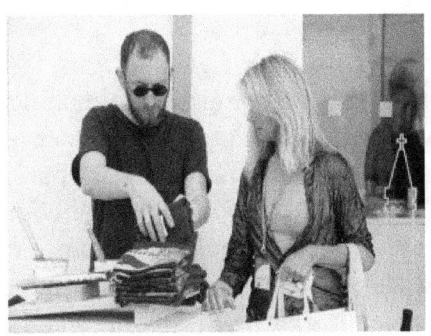

The day we make a stand and say, for example, "I am not an object. I feel you are invalidating my feelings", the reaction may not be a textbook re-evaluation of the relationship. If the person mocks our feelings and screams, "Oh so your 'feelings' are more important than my eternal suffering…" (fill in something they constantly complain about), these are signs we are dealing with a narcissist, especially if the reaction is extreme – nuclear even – involving insults, threats, hysteria, put-downs and attempts to get other family members on board to convince us (not them of course) to have therapy. Anyone who has been a doormat or family/social dustbin and who suddenly stands up and says, "No more" is likely to endure an intense outburst of wrath, since acceptance that we are in fact not an object would mean the narcissist would have to confront their real image, not the false one, and this they cannot do. In situations like this screaming back, hysteria and threatening is the worst possible reaction, since this will endorse their claim we are the one who's nuts. Let the difficult person have their enraged reaction, but if necessary we repeat our position in a calm, monotone voice (monotone to help us control our own emotions). No angry emails. Best course of action is immediate withdrawal and either ending the relationship or restricting it to practical matters. Our core values may have moved so far away from our original family/friends any extended contact is harmful and irritating to both sides. Rumination is likely, since there is no closure; distance is therefore the best possible option in order to distract us from harmful, stress-inducing thoughts. If abusive phone calls or nasty letters/emails arrive, we ignore them. Later, much later, introspection can be employed, in case anything (however minor) about what they said about us is true.

Rude strangers :

If a stranger is rude to us, without real reason and without knowing us from Adam, it is likely they are hard to live with and that it is nothing to do with us, so it is wise to say to ourselves, *I'm not going to take this personally*. However…difficult one, since in the heat of the moment, they do seem to be attacking *us*. Remaining Zen and not responding will perhaps limit conflict, but it is deeply unsatisfactory, since it will appear that the rude shop assistant/bank teller/tour guide etc. has "won". They have disrespected us without possible equalisation at a later stage. We can move away, but the balance has not been reestablished and as we do not know them, is unlikely ever to be. The injustice and souring of our mood is devilishly difficult to get rid of if we are unable to state our case. Best course of action, assuming the difficult stranger is not likely to physically attack us (in which case a disappearing act is advisable), is therefore to make one short but sharp retort, and then withdraw immediately. Here are two examples from real life :

On a plane, a young mother still carrying her pregnancy weight was struggling to put her suitcase in the overhead locker with two whiny toddlers. An impatient passenger behind her said, "If you weren't so fat you wouldn't be taking so long and holding everyone up." The mother counted to ten, turned to the passenger and, paraphrasing Winston Churchill said loudly, "I am fat and you are ugly. But I can go on a diet." Then she sat down and looked away to end the exchange.

At the pool an office worker in his fifties, trying to pack in a lunchtime swim, picked up a polystyrene board to swim with from a plastic crate – belonging to the pool – containing dozens of other boards. The aqua gym teacher slammed her foot on the man's hand and said, "I need those." The man looked at the twelve portly ladies cycling on the spot in the pool for a short while, each already with their board. There were obviously many spare boards so he tried again to extract one. The aqua gym teacher said, "I said no," in a very aggressive tone. The man let go the board and looked at the gym teacher saying, "Oh I'm so sorry. I can see you are a very aggressive person. Apologies, I should have noticed from those deep wrinkles on your upper lip that you have trouble controlling your negative emotions." He then entered the pool and back-stroked away. The entire gym class heard.

In both instances the exchange was brief, honest and calm, but emotions were equalised. No rumination ensued – at least not in the people defending themselves against the difficult person. Note in both of these cases the person attacked by the stranger paused to consider their reaction first and was therefore able to choose one for maximum effect.

Rude colleagues:

Two possibilities – either the colleague has power over us or he/she doesn't. If the colleague has no power (and is for example acting as though she does), then failure to react will lead to harmful rumination. After the statutory counting to ten, breathing deeply to avoid sounding angry (even though our heart may be racing), we make our response.

Example :

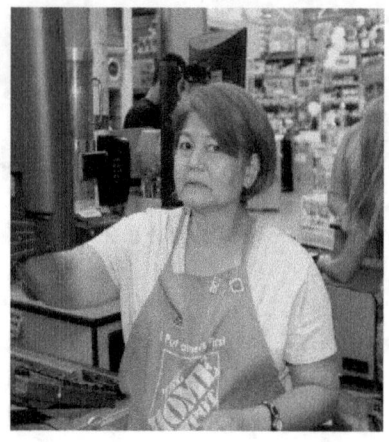

Rude colleague : "I can't believe you screwed up so badly there." Count to ten. Response to difficult colleague : "How interesting to see you also have an aggressive streak. Is this a new thing, or have I just uncovered it?" Ah yes, the skill of the put-down. To avoid souring the atmosphere at work – after all, we have to continue to work in it after the exchange is over – we use humour.

If the colleague does have power over us then silence and withdrawal is usually the best strategy, unless we are extremely good at the humorous but pointed response which will not challenge their authority. People in authority often got there because they wanted power over others. If we are fortunate enough to have a boss who took up the position in order to discover his or her inner demons and engage in 24/7 introspection, then a fairer exchange can take place, but let's face it...there ain't many of them about, and they aren't likely to be difficult people. Although it may lead to rumination, we won't regret silence in a case like this, whereas we may regret an impulsive angry response. And regrets, fear of consequences and belly-aching remorse are worse in triggering the stress response.

So in this case, the lesser of two evils unfortunately. And if it happens all the time, best to get away from that person if we can – change jobs/departments/activity – since it may be a vibrational personality clash. It is well known people behave differently depending on who they are with. One boss was particularly cruel and overbearing to a young girl who would tremble in fear whenever she was near him. In fact this was because he was rejected by a girl who strongly resembled her years back. Deep down it might not be about us at all, just the fact the difficult person in question is using us to exorcise their own hang-ups. There is a reason for their bad behaviour (but it doesn't mean it's not bad behaviour).

If the worst comes to the worst, "I can see you feel very strongly about this," is a good all-rounder. No one can object to our having said it, and it liberates us from having to swallow our bile. Let's drop the need to always be right with difficult people. The one-liner is enough. Conflict is necessary for growth. It expands consciousness and fosters appreciation of its opposite. Rumination, regrets and bitterness write themselves across our brows and add decades to our appearance. Developing high interpersonal intelligence means learning how to successfully deal with each individual person we encounter according to their temperament.

Dodgy Knees

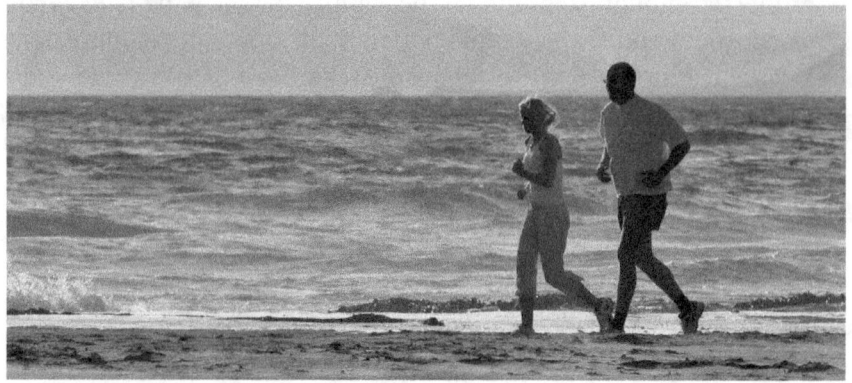

Anyone on a trip to the Austrian Alps will notice a large proportion of elderly walkers striding up the mountain, and fewer striding down. Taking the cable car down the mountain after walking up is something older people with dodgy knees go in for, since walking down steep paths can be more painful.

Many people will tell you that knee pain and arthritis in the knee joints are inevitable after middle age. The problem is that the cartilage that provides the padding in the knee wears out, and the bones start rubbing together, causing pain. Muscles also shrink in size by up to 40%, which means we lose strength. Losing this muscular support in later years makes us more likely to experience knee problems and to start to walk with bent knees, which is easier when the muscles are shorter and weaker, but makes us more likely to fall.

To make matters worse, the knee joint is one of the most complex ; the design compromise is between mechanical complexity and enormous power. It is more likely to be injured than any other joint in the body. Injuries can be caused by sport that combines running, jumping and stopping with quick changes of direction such as squash, football and skiing, as well as by accidents such as the dashboard injury in car accidents. A serious knee injury often leads to severe arthritis if no measures are taken to prevent decline.

Signs of a dodgy knee joint include :

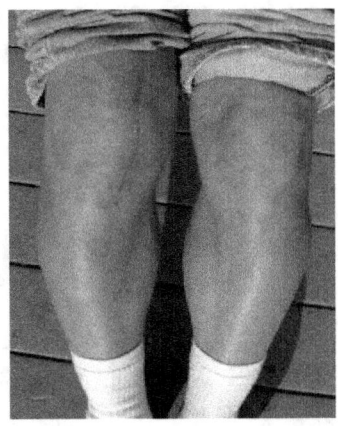

• Stiffness, difficulty in bending the knee
• Creaks and clicks
• Heat around the joint
• Swelling
• Pain
• Numbness

We often hear of people saying they used to go running but their knees can't take it any more. Distance running has often been seen as to blame for a busted knee. But recent studies have shown that there is little evidence to support this view. The reason for the confusion is that runners have more bone spurs than sedentary people their own age. A bone spur is a bump or growth that forms as the body tries to repair itself by building extra bone. It typically forms in response to pressure, rubbing or stress that continues over a long period of time. However, it turns out runners do not suffer from the wearing away of cartilage that normally accompanies bone spurs. Active people have greater cartilage volume than couch potatoes and therefore are less likely to suffer from painful arthritis as the bones grate against each other. Knee arthritis is therefore less common in people who exercise.

In a 2013 study (http://www.ncbi.nlm.nih.gov), adult runners, including many aged 45 or older, had a lower incidence of knee osteoarthritis and hip replacement than age-matched walkers, with the adults who accumulated the most mileage over the course of seven years having the lowest risk, possibly, the study's author speculated, because running improved the health of joint cartilage and kept them lean as they aged. Long distance running seems to have a protective effect. The only caveat is if an injury is already present, in which case the RICE method is advocated (rest, ice, compression and elevation).

If we want ageless knees, the medical advice now is to :

- Lose weight – increased rates of obesity have resulted in an epidemic of osteoarthritis.

- Exercise – as long as this is combined with periods of warming up, cooling off and rest. The right exercise has both a preventative and curative effect.

Knee problems are not inevitable with age. Children and teenagers are just as likely to experience knee pain if they participate in activities that require repetitive movements. If we take good care of our knees before there is a problem we can really help ourselves. Without healthy knees there is no independence, and our physical world shrinks. The time and effort spent on avoiding rickety joints pays huge dividends over the years. It is not true that knee problems are inevitable as we age – most people do not have knee pain. Let us take steps to ensure we stay pain-free.

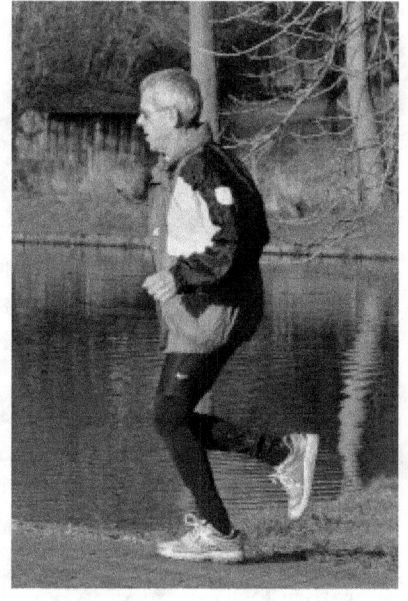

Apples and Pears – beating middle age spread

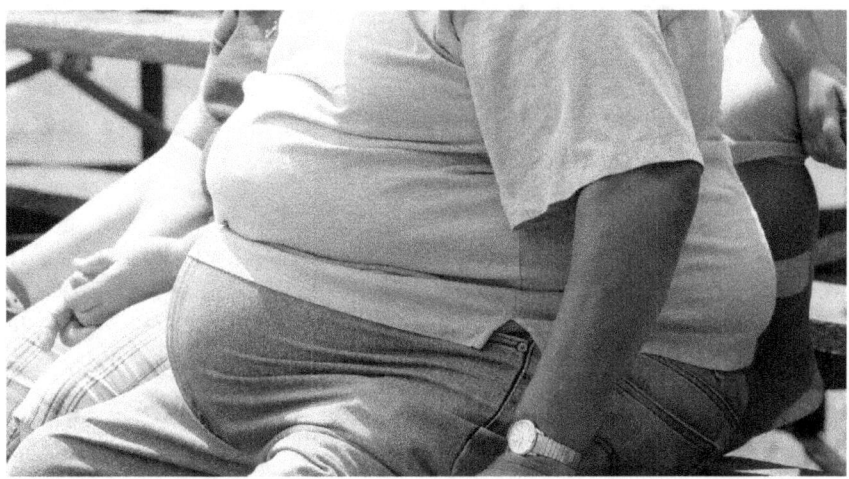

Theresa did a twirl in her new sharp suit. "When I hit fifty I assumed the weight was piling on because that is what happens in middle age. When I hit sixty I realised I was kidding myself, and stopped eating as much. That's how I got into this outfit."

It is easy to adopt a "ho hum" attitude to a bulging midriff in middle age, since everyone around us is similar and it seems this is just what happens when we get older. The drop in testosterone that men experience (but see page 90) plus high insulin and a fatty liver can mean a big belly and man-boobs, and women lose estrogen and therefore have proportionally more testosterone, so fat shifts from the bottom and thighs to the abdomen; this is how women who were always naturally slim find they can no longer eat what they like. Don't look at your thin legs, it's your midriff that can cause problems. But did Nature actually mean us to get all the health problems that come with middle age spread?

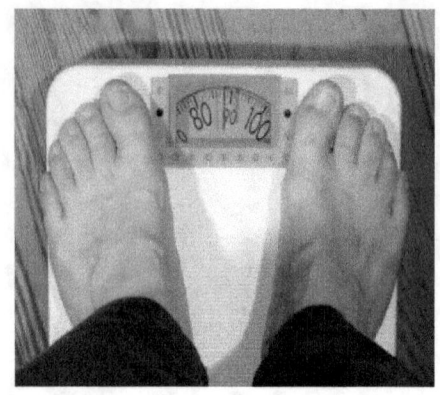

A waistline of more than 35in (89cm) for women and 40in (102cm) for men leads to a substantially increased risk of heart disease and type-2 diabetes.

Fat around the abdomen raises blood pressure and cholesterol. It increases the risk of diabetes, Alzheimer's and some cancers. Fat that forms around our vital organs is called visceral fat and sends out its own chemical messages, unlike subcutaneous fat. It causes inflammation in the blood vessels which can lead to cardio-vascular disease and calcium deposits which harden the arteries.

Middle age spread is the worst possible type of fat we can get. Pear-shapes become apple-shapes, the classic walking heart attack cases. And let's face it: it's ageing to our appearance – it looks pretty awful.

Remedies? Weight training as well as exercise can keep an expanding waistband in check.

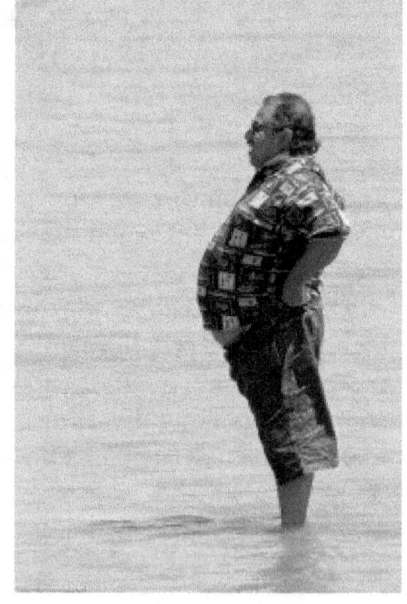

No more excuses: middle age spread is not natural, and those around us who got fat after forty are playing dice with their health. Fatigue is due to a lack of exercise, not the other way round. Lack of exercise decreases muscle mass, which reduces the number of calories burnt : vicious circle.

Hormonal changes and a more sedentary lifestyle mean that we cannot carry on eating three square meals a day in middle age like we did when we were younger. If we do, prepare the route to the outsize shop. There's no two ways about it : we have to eat less.

How normal is middle age spread? Answer : not normal at all. Unless you believe illness and being a blob is Nature's gift to the middle aged, now is the time for action. Our body is our machine: if we don't take care of it, no one else will.

Is an unhappy marriage better than none?

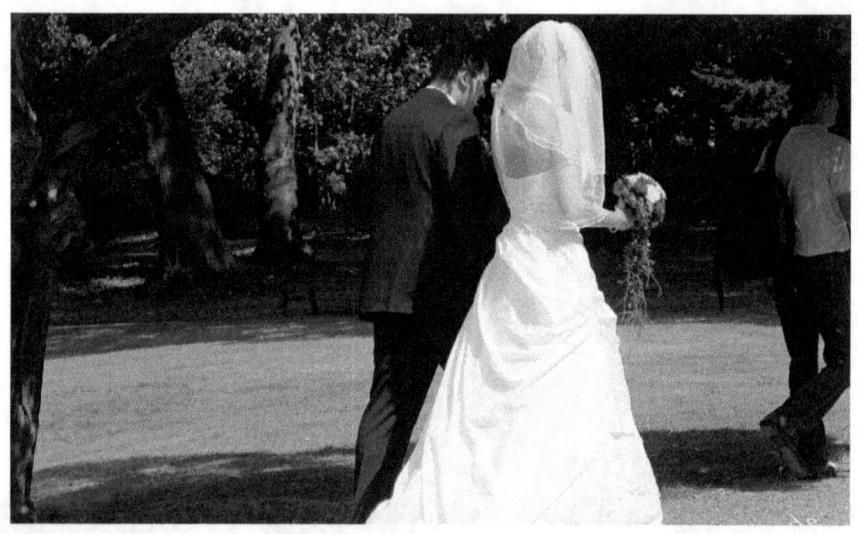

Some studies have shown that marital happiness has no effect on the benefits of being married. This is clearly absolute nonsense. Any statistical health advantage in unhappy marriages almost certainly comes from women telling men to see a doctor when something seems wrong. But emotional stress and an unsatisfactory relationship is clearly going to impact health. Healthy relationships increase lifespan. Abusive, violent, manipulative, exploitative relationships are ruinous to health.

"I can't understand why my father died at 72," said Sandy. "He jogged every day, was a non-smoking vegetarian and did yoga every morning. He never reacted angrily when my mother called him names and bullied him, he was one of the most placid men I know, so he didn't even fit the Type A profile."

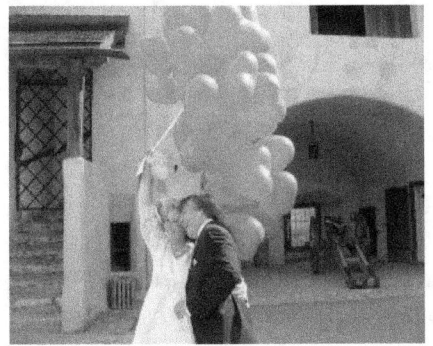

Marital stress is associated with thickening of the heart chamber (unlike job stress), elevated levels of adrenaline, high blood pressure and the production of cytokines which cause inflammation (a newly recognised cardiac risk).

However some studies appear to show that divorce can damage one's physical health so dramatically that the person never recovers. Oh please! The end of a high-stress, unloving, possibly abusive relationship will immediately cause cortisol and adrenaline levels to sink as fear, unpredictability and constant repression of one's own needs and desires disappear. It is often a matter of urgency that man should put asunder what God has joined together, and while we're on the subject what is the point of a very long life lived in an unhappy marriage? There is no prize waiting at the finishing line.

There is no marriage contract detector in our genes; rather it is a social convention that being bound together under law – law is also not a biological feature – is stabilising. It is our perception that marriage is stable that reassures us. But for many people marriage is destabilising – especially people with depressed, aggressive, unloving, unfaithful, manipulative or personality-disordered spouses. The only factor causing illness in divorce from partners such as these is guilt and the feeling of failure, again coming straight out of our own thinking. Children raised in abusive and dysfunctional

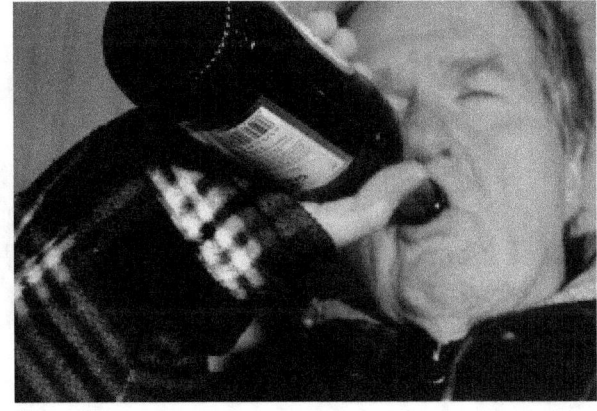

families will be more damaged than if they live with one loving parent. Lundy Bancroft in his book *Why Does He Do That?* reports that the men he treated for domestic abuse were men who witnessed their father abusing their mother. "I'm so afraid that divorcing my husband will damage my daughters," said one woman, who had discovered her husband had been unfaithful dozens of times, including with women she thought were friends. But the opposite is true: a woman who does not love herself enough to change a life like that will model an unhealthy pattern of relationships to her daughters.

This isn't rocket science.

A relationship should last only as long as it serves the people in it – emotionally, not financially. For those who prefer the marriage bond, we need a new set of vows – not until death do us part, but as long as the relationship benefits us both. There are few benefits in getting married these days – pension rights and the next-of-kin status are some of the remaining legal perks – but many people feel these are insufficient to compensate for the legal fees and sense of failure if people wish to become unmarried, nor do they counterbalance the tendency to stop making an effort with each other once you have nabbed your man/woman which is so often the case within a legal bond. There are few things advocating involving the State in one's love life, and many reasons for not doing so.

Marriage certainly does not protect against boredom, strife, stress, abuse or infidelity – it never did. It does not protect children from emotional abandonment, and children's happiness comes from empathetic and supportive parents, not from a legal institution.

A happy marriage is a wonderful way to live one's life, but it is this word "happy" that these longevity studies so often leave out. Marriage is never more important than the people in it. Being married has nothing to do with life extension. Being happy does.

Resolving the pain of loss

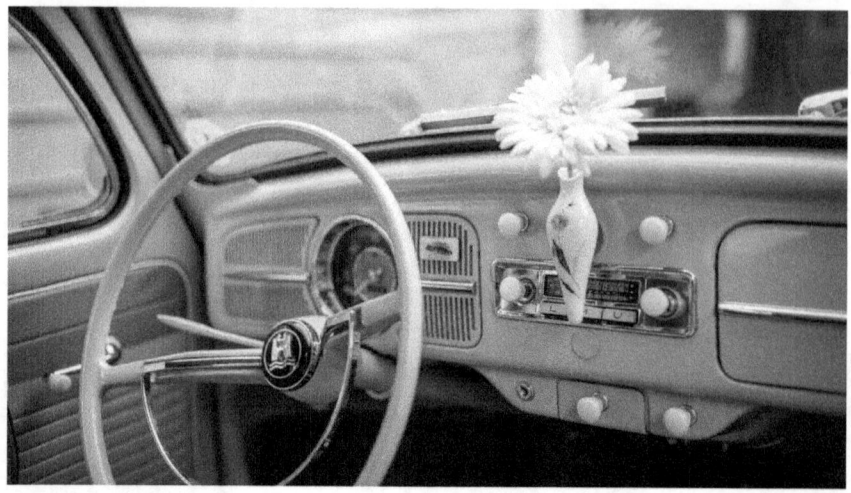

People say that when they lose a loved friend or family member, part of them dies too. Perhaps they don't realise what they are saying, but in feeling this way they are conditioning themselves to follow in their footsteps. If we were not surrounded by more and more of our acquaintances passing away as our life progresses, the possibility of extended life would etch itself into our cells. Put differently, it is the death of other people that deprives us of the possibility of long life.

We must learn to deal with loss and change if we are to stay ageless. The loss of our past – the familiar buildings that are now gone, the people who once staffed services we use, the relatives we used to meet in summer or New Year – shocks us into thinking we are on our way out too. The subliminal messages our emotions send to us say : *if the building is gone, then what am I still doing here?*

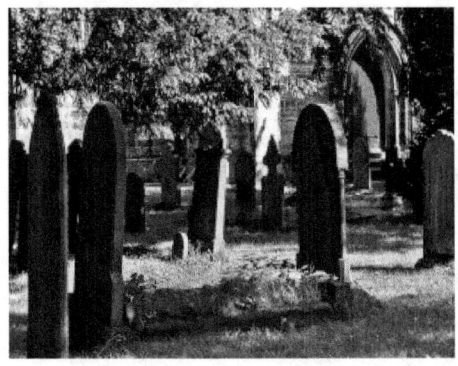 Feelings of nostalgia and yearning for an earlier period while complaining about the present are the hallmark of the middle-aged and beyond. It hurts us to see the world changing so quickly. But it is only by embracing change, allowing it, and saluting those who pass from this world with a gentle acceptance that we can sit comfortably in each new epoch, and thus allow our lives to flourish in them. Refusing to learn how to use new systems, doggedly doing things the old way is walking along the highway towards infirmity and obsolescence.

Perhaps the greatest challenge comes with the death of a parent. The most likely age of an adult child on the death of a parent is between 45 and 64 years of age. Since we learnt how to do most things from our parents, if they die at a certain age we may feel condemned to do the same. If we exceed their age of death we think we are living on borrowed time. Becoming an adult orphan often coincides with the shock that most people on this earth are now younger than us. How can this be, this was never the case before?! We may conclude the world has become hostile towards us, and that we no longer belong in it. This is relinquishing power over our health and destiny. It is sending a poisonous e-mail to our cells.

This is not about denial. Denial is said to be one of the stages of mourning, but there is no typical response to loss. Dr Kübler-Ross who spoke of the five stages of grief said herself there is no imperative need to pass through each of them, and even less so if we have thought through the meaning of death and the possibility of controlling our lifespan. Instead this is about taking control.

One aspect of the death of a parent that is more often than not suppressed is the feeling of relief, and release. Common though it is, fear that it is disrespectful prevents people from speaking of it openly. Freedom to be ourselves fully is a sensation many bereaved "children" have experienced, which can mean we only fully become an adult in late middle age. With no one to please and no one's disapproval to fear, we are free to choose the paths that attract us. "When she died," said Jean of her mother's death, "her power over me was finally gone. I felt free to be successful at last, and no longer had to fear her envy." The secret to living beyond 80 – 90 years is to find a way to reconcile the unresolved hurt of losing the things and people we love. We are answerable ultimately only towards ourselves. Loss is a part of the process of change and renewal. It never stopped, we only notice it more as we accumulate more years and experience. We need to allow other people their experience of death without taking it personally. This is love without attachment, unconditional love that is not about what we

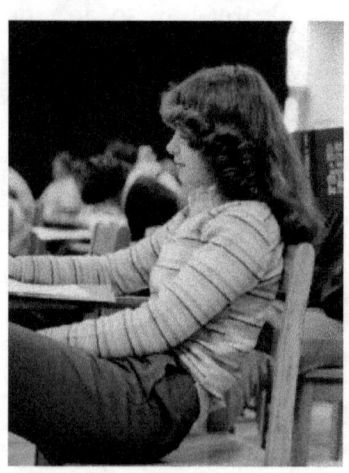

can get from other people. Loss is part of the ebb and flow of the earth's energy, it is a force for good since it allows new forms and new ideas to emerge. It should never frighten us into feeling our time is past and that our demise is fast approaching. Just as the doctrine of reincarnation has us adopting many guises and roles from one life to another, whoever stays ageless does the same, but within a single lifespan.

Rasputin

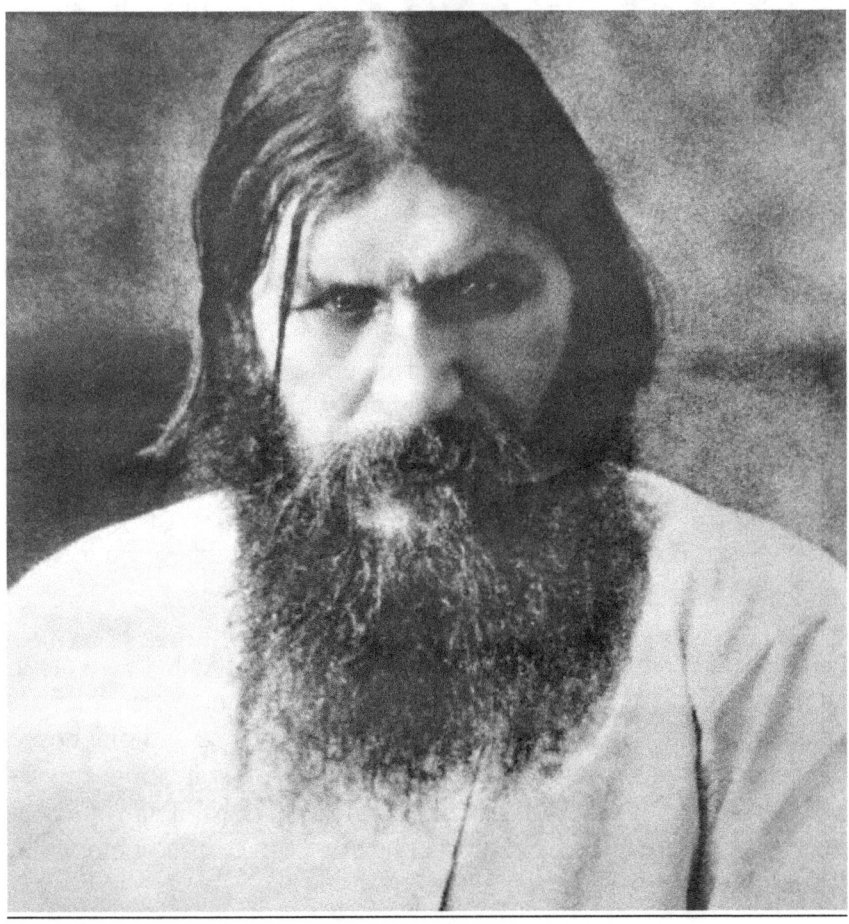

Rasputin is one of the handful of historical figures who seemingly possessed a superhuman life force. He is famous for having been particularly difficult to kill, and his unusual gifts as a mystic and healer are often cited as the reason why he came close to achieving immortality.

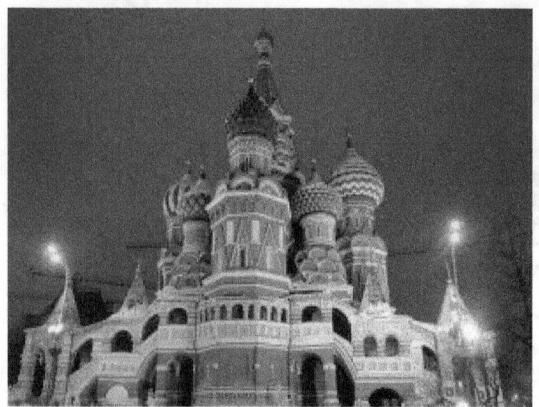

He was not an educated man but he underwent a religious transformation during a three month stay in a monastery at the age of 18, and although he married and had children, he began a life as a wandering holy man. He was notorious for having a magnetic effect on women. Boney M's classic song has made him go down in history as a sleaze ball of gargantuan proportions, given to drunkenness and orgies, the lover of the Russian queen, a goatish conman with an enormous wart on his penis that made women pass out cold during orgasm. Others claim he was a victim of anti-tsarist propaganda spread by the communists, and that he was genuinely saintly and a mystic with phenomenal powers. Many Russians think he should be canonised.

He survived the first attempt on his life in 1914 when a woman attacked him with a knife crying, "I have killed the antichrist", causing his entrails to spill out. She was imprisoned and diagnosed as insane, but following surgery he survived. His healing powers came to the attention of the tsars, and unlike any of the medical men who had tried to treat the young prince Alexei's hemophilia, Rasputin was able to help the boy.

Felix Yusupov, a Russian prince and friend of the Romanov tsars, wrote a book from exile in Paris in the 1920s in which he described the events of the 29th December 1916. Exasperated at Rasputin's influence over the emperor and his wife, a plot was hatched by courtiers to assassinate Rasputin. In the book Felix Yusupov claims Rasputin was invited to his palace on the pretext of healing his wife Irina. He was instructed to wait in a lounge, where pastries and wine laced with cyanide awaited him. Rasputin seemed to hesitate before eating them, but although the cyanide was enough to kill five men, his only reaction on swallowing them was salivation and burping. Rasputin asked Yusupov to play the guitar and sing. For two hours this "nightmare" continued. When Yusupov checked in with his co-conspirators he was pale with despair, saying that Rasputin had eaten and drunk the poisoned food and nothing had happened.

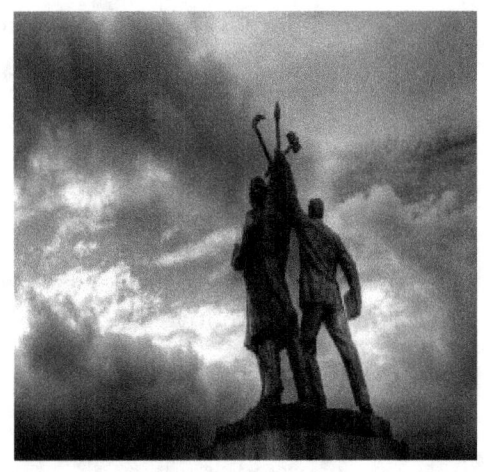

Yusupov records that when the cyanide failed to kill Rasputin, he decided to end it and shoot him in the back while Rasputin was admiring a decorative cross. At first Rasputin fell to the floor, but when Yusupov returned Rasputin revived, grabbed him by the neck and fled into the snow. Yusupov shot him again, missed, and bit himself in the wrist to make himself concentrate, then shot Rasputin again in the head. He then beat him repeatedly with a dumbbell, and Yusupov and his co-conspirators tied him up with rope and dumped the body in the river. At some point they also castrated him. When the body was found floating downstream, his hands were in a raised position, causing speculation he was still alive under the ice and was trying to get the rope off his hands.

Modern-day mystics ask:

Could Rasputin, as a mystic, have been told the secrets of tantra at the monastery, channelling the energy of his many lovers to build an extremely powerful life force? Could Rasputin have exercised some control over his reality, as manifest in his healing powers? In the movie *The Matrix*, when Neo realises his mind and his thoughts are creating the world around him, the bullets have no power to kill him.

Rasputin was buried in secret to avoid desecration, but some have claimed Rasputin was the legendary Count of St Germain, the immortal who appears periodically at times of crisis in earth's history.

The sceptics claim :

- Yusupov deliberately missed because the transvestite prince was in love with the monk.
- The autopsy showed no cyanide in the body, only alcohol. Rasputin did not touch the poisoned food and drink.
- Historians have suggested Yusupov's version is grossly exaggerated or falsified.
- Rasputin was buried in Imperial Park, but dug up by revolutionaries in 1917 and burnt in a forest.

Whatever the truth, Rasputin has gone down in history as a "mad monk" who was almost indestructible. Before he died, if indeed he did die, he was poisoned, shot four times, clubbed, castrated, exposed to freezing conditions and drowned. On his last day on earth he was 47. It is interesting to speculate how long he would have lived if he had not made so many enemies.

Help my unbelief...

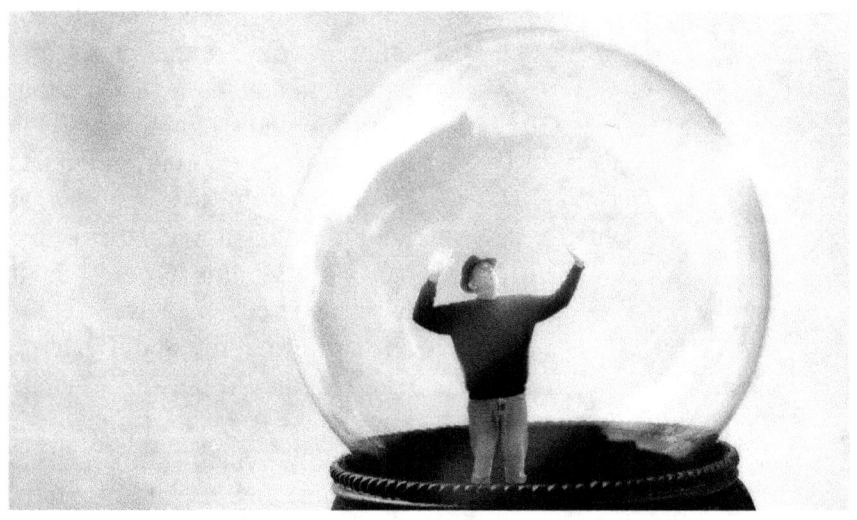

The placebo effect has been known about for centuries, and is the basis for the success of medical quackery and peddlers of snake oil. Prescribing a pill, or surgery even, that has no actual effect while telling the patient it has, will alleviate symptoms in over a third of patients. Some doctors believe the placebo effect is purely psychological, that although the patient believes he has improved, he hasn't at all. This view claims the response is a result of conditioning where patients have come to expect an improvement after taking medication.

The problem with this theory is that research shows that the improvements experienced by subjects on a placebo are measurable. A study was done in 2002 at UCLA on a group of patients with depression. Those receiving a placebo who had reported feeling better demonstrated an even greater amount of positive brain activity than those on the drug, and in places the drug did not reach. Placebos are also thought to trigger the release of endorphins, causing the sensation of pain to decrease. It is clear then that the belief of the subject has a direct physical effect on the body.

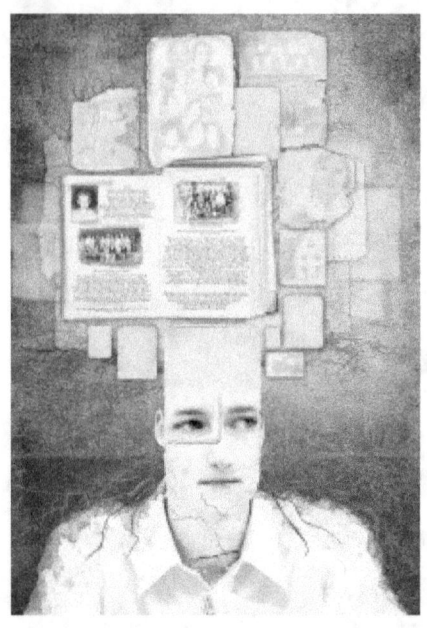

Beliefs about what it is to be old come to us through a filter of other people's experiences and expectations. If we accept that infirmity and death around 80 is inevitable, every time new facts come to light to support that belief, we assimilate them. We can observe this process as it happens every time we receive new information about ageing or about an old person someone knows. If someone or something – such as this book – calls these beliefs into question, we may reject them if they do not fit what we have accepted as true. The beliefs of a society provide a blueprint for what it becomes – this is most obvious in the creation of parallel societies of immigrants, or ghetto-isation, where migrants who have left their home societies for a new life recreate the society they left behind, even becoming fossilised versions of it while their country of origin has moved on.

The power of belief is what underpins the claim that faith can move mountains. When Jesus healed someone in the gospels, over and over again he attributes it to that person's belief: the woman in the crowd healed from hemorrhaging – 'your faith has made you well' – the two blind men following Jesus – 'do you believe that I can do this?' – the blind beggar on the road to Jericho – 'your faith has healed you'. He did no miracles in Nazareth because of the people's unbelief.

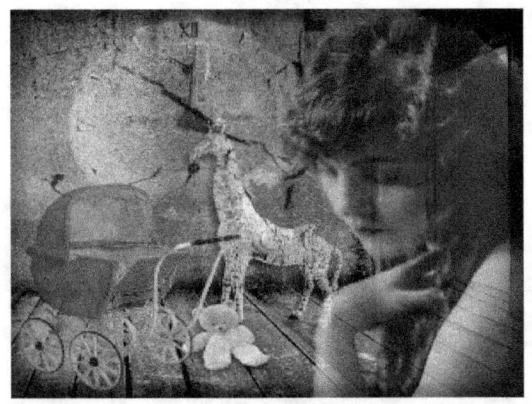

Our beliefs and convictions come from experience, sometimes from our earliest experiences, and are soaked in the emotions which surrounded those experiences so that picking the beliefs apart can be painful and difficult. "I still recall a boy calling me a fat cow and to go on a diet," said Margaret. "I'm sure he's forgotten, but I can describe everything about that classroom even today 50 years on." At a very deep level we can believe we are unattractive, unintelligent or uninteresting. Few people question the strong impact of experience on convictions such as these, but almost no one extends the idea to areas such as our health and how we age.

Our beliefs affect our appearance. If we think we look old we will. If we buy into the archetype of "fifty", "sixty" or "eighty", imprinted on our mind by hundreds of people who reached that age before us, our physical appearance will adjust to reflect that archetype. We must not underestimate the power of the spirit beneath the flesh – it has been documented again and again that the minute the soul left the body, the corpse no longer resembled the person who once inhabited it.

Our beliefs – as documented by the placebo effect – also affect our physical condition. For this reason it is imperative that we use affirmations – quietly to ourselves and also in conversation with others – to gain mastery over our bodies. Examples of this are saying, "I had backache earlier on but it's getting better now," (even if it's not) rather than, "If this gets any worse I'm going to have to take the day off," (encouraging poor health in oneself to obtain something desirable). We can affirm, "The diagnosis for this disease is poor but fortunately I am in the percentage likely to overcome it," (even if we have no idea whether statistics actually back us up, which doesn't matter since they are only statistics!). This is taking control.

We cannot change the things that others have created in the world we live in, but we can change the things we believe about the world so that it rearranges itself into one more fitting someone who stays ageless.

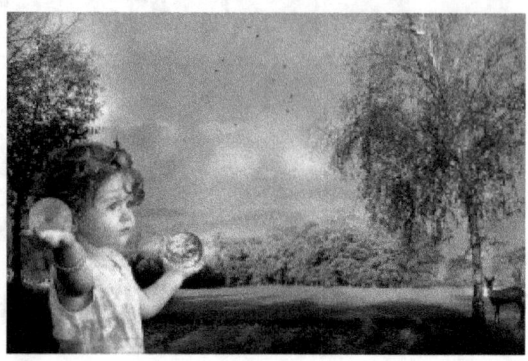

Martin Luther King once said that every man must do two things alone : his own believing and his own dying. Let us make sure this is true for us.

Mutant Ninja Worms

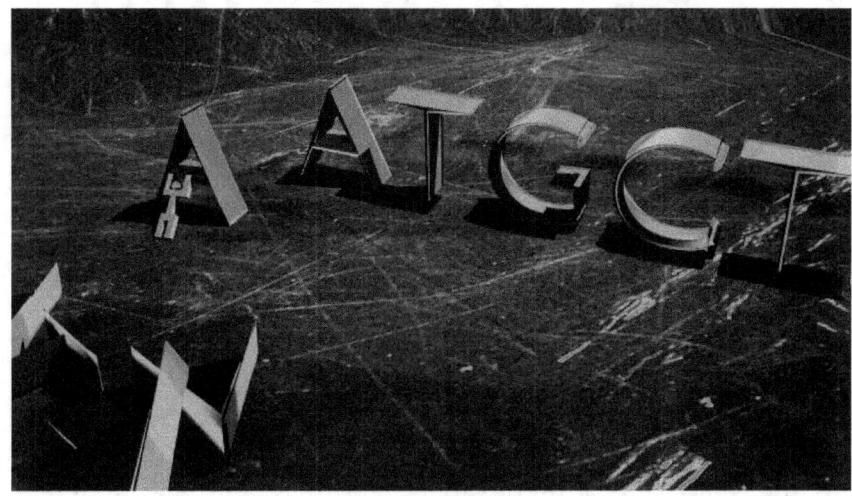

Throughout the last century there was a rather passive attitude to ageing. It was assumed that we just wear out, though it was known that rates of ageing were in part at least regulated by genes, since different species have such different lifespans. Rats and squirrels are the same size for example but live 3 and 25 years respectively. Scientist Cynthia Kenyon has carried out research to determine which genes govern ageing, and to do so chose a simple organism with a short lifespan – the C elegans worm. It was found that there was a mutant version of the worm with a longer lifespan. Those worms showing very low activity of a gene known as Daf-2 had double the lifespan and also aged more slowly. At 13 days normal worms looked old, and moved sluggishly. The longer lived mutants were much healthier and as active as very young worms.

Daf-2 is a gene that specifies the genetic code for a hormone receptor similar to the receptor for insulin and IGF-1. The function of this receptor is to speed up ageing. Therefore worms with low

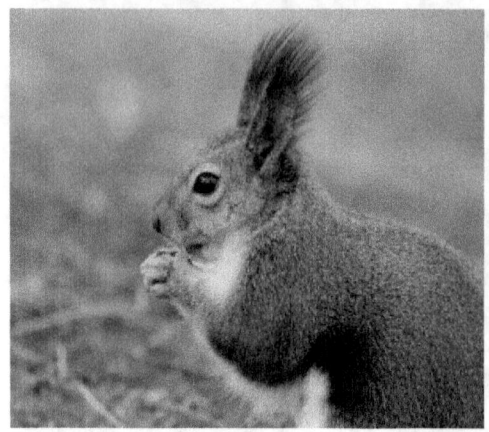

Daf-2 activity age more slowly. In order for low Daf-2 activity mutants to live long, another gene known as Daf-16 has to be active. For this reason it is known as the sweet 16 gene.

Why does low insulin and low IGF-1 receptor activity lead to long life?

One theory is that it is a response to the environment. In a favourable environment there is normal growth and metabolism, which is promoted by insulin/IGF-1 signalling. In a harsh environment there is little food and thus low insulin/IGF-1 signalling. Danger! Danger! is the message being sent to the organism. In response animals activate Daf-16 which sends a protective response to the body's cells. Insulin receptor activity drops – it does not stop altogether (which would be fatal) but slows down, and this extends lifespan. The fantastic thing is that not only does it lengthen the organism's life but it also makes it resistant to practically anything – in the case of the worm this means oxidative stress, heat, pathogens, hypoxia, heavy metals etc. Even better, the same response that protects the worm from this list of external stressors makes it equally resistant to its own internal stress (metabolic rather than psychological stress one imagines in a microscopic worm, but it is tempting to imagine the implications for humans).

So, does this research only apply to C elegans? Research has already established that inhibiting genes encoding the insulin or IGF-1 receptors can extend lifespan in mice but there is some evidence for humans too. A study of centenarian Ashkenazi Jews found they were more likely to have a reduction of the function of the IGF-1 receptors than those who died earlier. Humans have three different Daf-16-like genes. One is FOXO 3A. Humans seem to be susceptible to the same mutations in the gene as our famous worm. Variations in human DNA can affect its activity. These variations are associated with exceptional longevity all over the world.

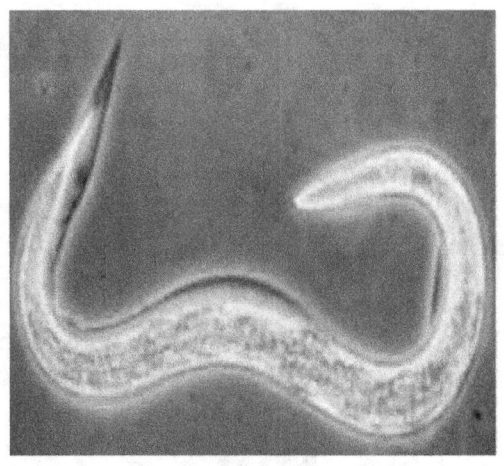

Whether we have the mutant genes or not, the point here is triggering low insulin and IGF-1 receptor activity. The way to do this is to create a harsh external environment - i.e. a famine. In other words, restrict our calories, but be undernourished and not malnourished to avoid damaging our bodies in the process. If C elegans is given sugar (its diet is normally bacteria), it dies earlier. Glucose shortens lifespan. If we can't restrict calories, we should at least try and restrict sugar. The current recommended dose is 25g a day. Sometimes it is better therefore to buy full fat products, which may contain less sugar than the low fat versions.

__Too old to change?__

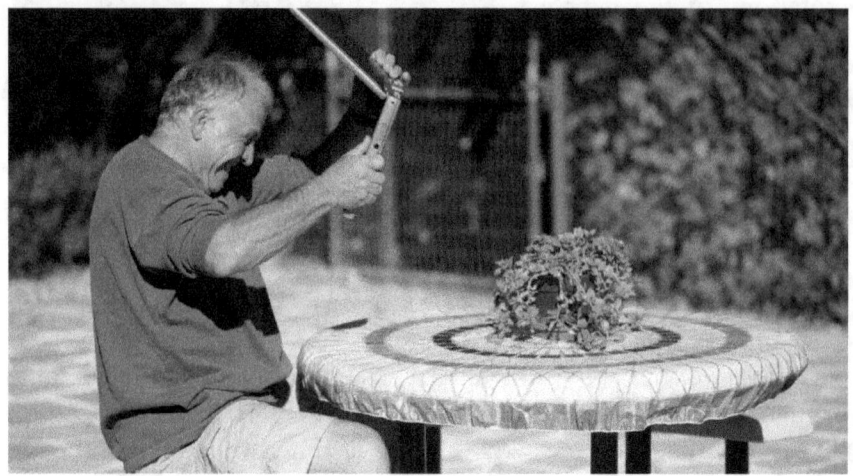

Our grandmothers were sometimes afraid of the telephone. Having grown up in a time when having one was a luxury, being expected to pick up that blasted thing that could suddenly start ringing out of the blue and then talk to it (!) was a source of some degree of stress.

Our mothers wring their hands over email and online forms. Even the phone book is online these days, you can't even make a decent phone call without having to switch on the computer.

And what about us? For many of us, Facebook, Twitter and all the even newer forms of social media are the equivalent of the phone and computer to the generations before us. The reaction to new ways of doing things is often far from enthusiastic. *If it ain't broke don't fix it*, we complain, *why change things when everything worked so well*? Our inner Luddite rails at the world, and just can't see the point of all this mindless online chatter. And there is a lot of truth in the criticism voiced by the older generation. Doing everything via a screen has distanced the younger generation from the deep satisfaction of reading a physical book, from the hidden joys contained in a shelf at the library, from the wisdom of slowing down and not communicating with anyone for a day, a weekend, a week....

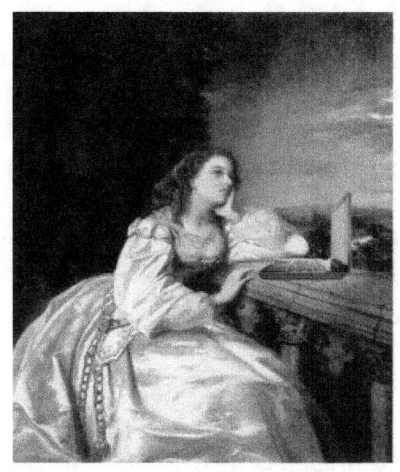

The problem is that if we constantly refuse to learn how to use new methods of social discourse we are aligning ourselves with a period of earth's history that is on its way out. "I don't know why they had to change to these irritating digital photocopiers," a secretary said. "The older ones worked just as well, didn't need to be programmed, and anyway I'm too old to change."

However, children resist change too, when it doesn't suit them, but they are less likely to complain when new ideas are introduced, and the reason is probably simply because they do not have to unlearn several old methods first, unlike adults, so it requires less effort.

Are older adults too old to change then? Is there any truth in the idea that older people should not be expected to learn new things?

Actually, there isn't. The adult brain is remarkably resilient. It seems to be capable of rewiring itself well into late middle age and beyond, incorporating new and different approaches into decades of experience. Not only does the middle-aged mind maintain many of the abilities of youth, but it also acquires new ones, possessing enduring potential for plasticity according to cognitive neuroscientist Patricia Reuter-Lorenz PhD of the University of Michigan in Ann Arbor. Older adults are also more positive and more able to sort through social situations. Some middle-agers even have *improved* cognitive abilities.

Researchers suspect that one reason middle-aged people are more resilient is that their brains have learned to accentuate the positive and eliminate the negative. Researchers at the University of Wisconsin found that in younger adults the amygdala, the brain's emotional 'nut', was activated when they looked at upsetting as well as 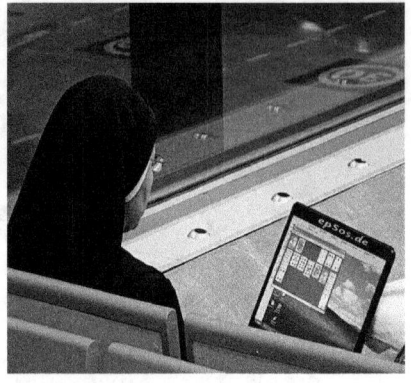 uplifting images. Adults in their middle and upper decades, by contrast, seemed to have the ability to screen out or dampen down negative emotions; their amygdalas lit up when they saw positive images but tended to ignore disturbing ones.

Most of us were brought up with the idea our brains start to die off practically the moment we are born, but this is not true. Neurons continue to grow in the cerebral cortex throughout life. Learning new skills (even something as banal as brushing our teeth with the other hand) can help 'fix' these new neurons in the brain, as can education – a degree appears to slow the brain's ageing process by up to a decade, adding a new twist to the cost-benefit analysis of higher education – and it is never too late to start educating oneself.

Problems older people encounter such as memory failure turn out to be not due to age but due to the diseases that often arise in later life such as diabetes (twice as likely to have memory problems) and high blood pressure (twice as likely to have areas of brain damage). Maintaining a vigorous exercise programme can help us avoid these medical conditions and thus make full use of the superior minds we develop the longer we stick around on the planet.

The Observer Effect

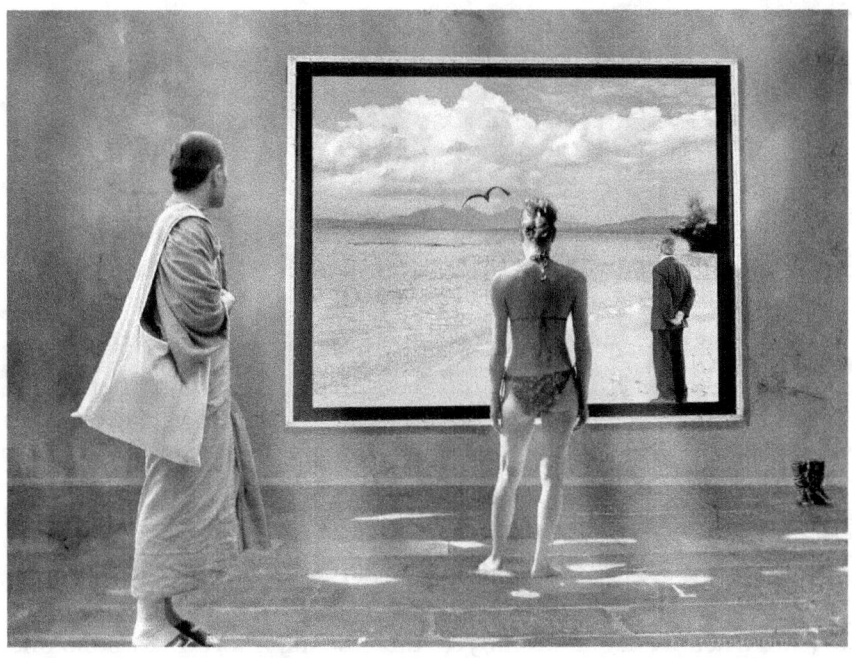

Most people interested in spirituality have heard of the strange property of electrons in an atom. The electrons are like a series of circular waves pulsating around the nucleus, occupying all possible positions at once, rather like ripples spreading out from a stone thrown into water. Only when a conscious observer tries to measure their position do they feel obliged to adopt one. Another analogy is that of a swarm of bees, that are all actually the same bee, until you try and focus on one.

If quantum physics is correct, the observer has a role in how the universe looks. Scientist and author Gregg Braden gives the example of scientists looking for the smallest particle in existence; he suggests they will never find it, since every time someone looks

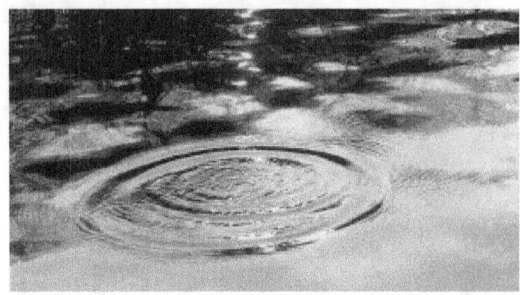 for something even smaller than the current smallest subatomic particle, the act of looking will call it into existence.

The question is, does the observer effect also occur at a macro, rather than just a micro level; does observing the universe call our everyday lives and events into existence?

Conventional science currently states that the observer effect does not apply to real life outside the lab, and anyone who suggests it does is guilty of quantum woo (or quantum BS). There is no proof it *doesn't* apply to real life either though. One might adopt a Pascal's Wager approach here : it might be better to assume that the observer effect does apply to real life until solid proof is found one way or the other, since if it is true it won't be too late to take control of our health and ageing when science 'catches up' (and if it isn't true, we'll have enjoyed the ride far more than someone getting depressed about their inevitable decline).

Every year we look for signs of ageing. Be aware that the act of looking might call those signs into existence. We must not just hope we will stay youthful, but believe it. Staying ageless is our default assumption, our set point, our basic belief. Saying, wow I look so much younger than last week every time we look in the mirror is an act of creation. If the general belief that ageing is inevitable is wrong, but we buy into it, how powerful is that belief?

The Staying Ageless experiment is this : We are part of the universal field. Thoughts are powerful, emotions more so – our heart's electric field is 500 times stronger than the brain's. Feeling we are young with our heart locks the bee into place. Believing we will not become old and infirm creates that reality.

Worth a try?

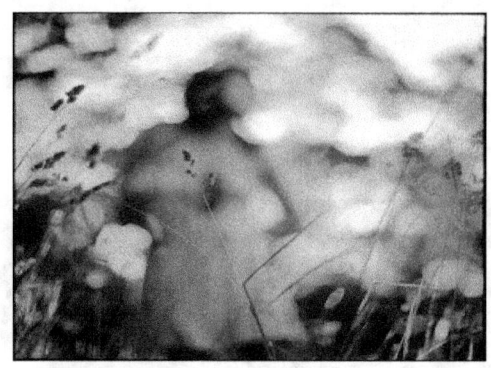

<u>Three Things</u>

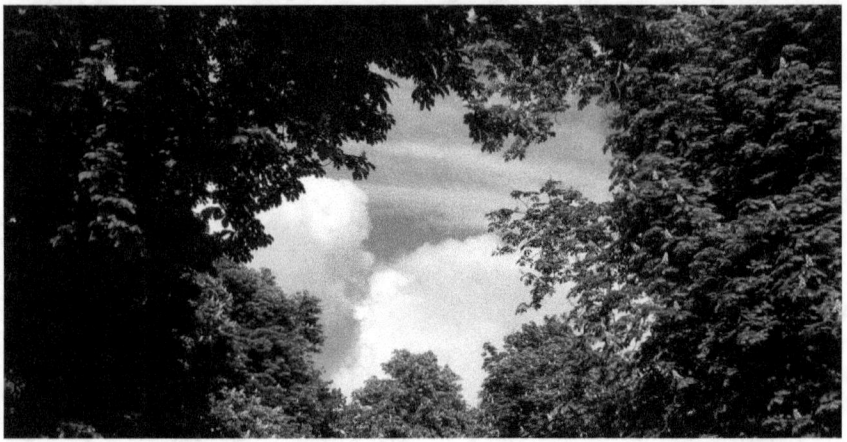

The Staying Ageless community is a group of individuals in countries all over the globe who are experimenting with mindfulness and lifestyle, in an attempt to determine to what extent ageing is a learned response. We have faith, even though this is a path few have trodden in the past. We have faith even though we may be mocked as deluded, arrogant, vain and even nuts. Faith, said St Paul, is the substance of things hoped for, the evidence of things not yet seen. It is our conviction that our lives will be a testament to these things so that they will indeed be seen. Staying Ageless is a lifestyle that involves countless aspects of our minds and bodies, but if we had to choose just three things that will ensure that we stay youthful, fit, bright and energetic all our lives, they are these:

1. Calorie restriction
2. Stress management
3. Belief

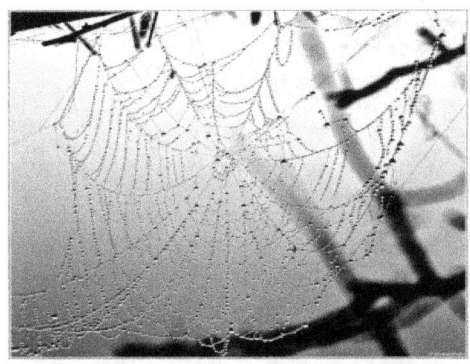

Calorie restriction acts on our cells, reducing toxins and minimising DNA damage due to oxidative stress caused by metabolising food. Stress management does not deny stress, but is aware of its effects, and uses it to kick-start the body into repair mode by quickly recovering from stressful experiences – physical activity or mental anguish – through mindfulness, meditation, music and monitoring thoughts.

Belief locks into the quantum brain, the field around us and within us, the interconnected web of life; it controls the matrix by exploiting the observer effect, according to which what we perceive creates reality. Having faith that we are still young and healthy, believing that ageing is caused by social conditioning, keeping the faith that ageing can be reversed is the most important factor of staying ageless.

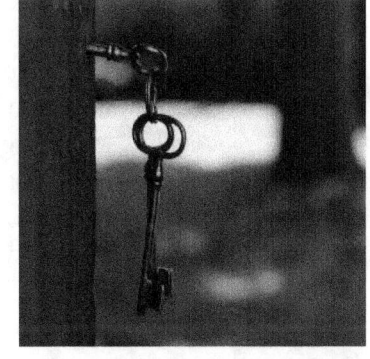

"And now these three remain: calorie restriction, stress management and faith. But the greatest of these is faith."

Photo Credit: ZeePack via Compfight cc
Photo Credit: jenny downing via Compfight cc

__Introspection__

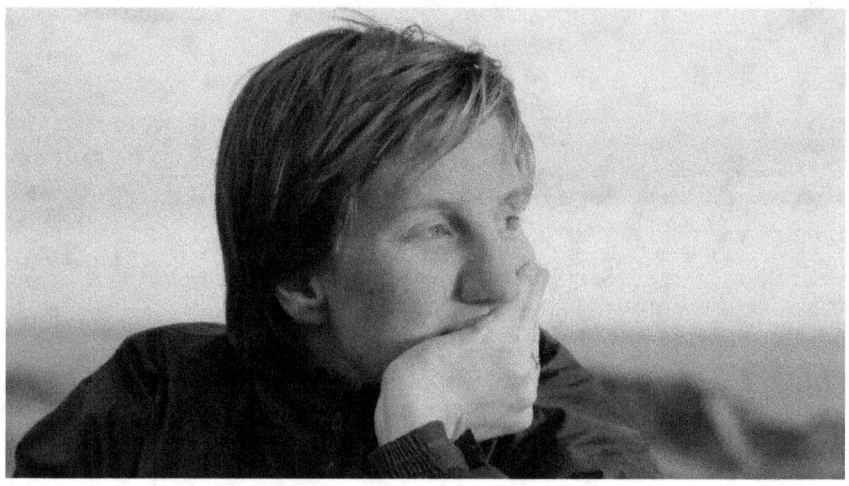

Very few people in the general population regularly engage in critical introspection. The ability to assess one's external behaviour against one's inner state is one of the habits followed by successful people – successful meaning happy, not just in money terms – and although in theory it is actually very easy, in practice it takes years to develop and requires constant maintenance to avoid slipping back into the view that the world has it in for us.

Introspection is the examination of our thoughts and feelings, the retrospective assessment of our behaviour and motives with the aim of either repeating successful moments or avoiding unfortunate ones in the future. It is not the same as external observation, whether this be impassive or critical of others. If it condemns flaws in others, it does so with the sole purpose of detecting the same flaw in ourselves.

Research suggests most people practise introspection around 5% of the time. This low figure comes from studies using beepers. Whenever the beeper went off, subjects were asked to record their thoughts. Self-aware thinking amounted to 5% of the time. The rest? Planning, complaining, thinking of the past, and criticising others, as well as structured thinking in connection with a task or job.

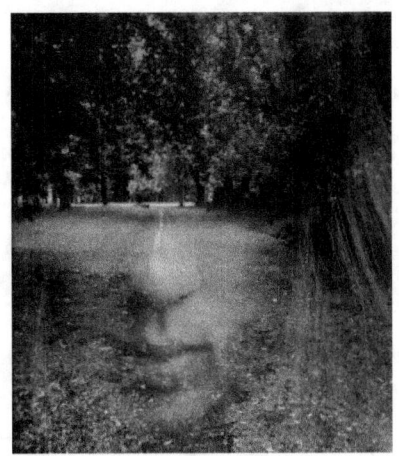

Most people, when faced with a problem, look outside themselves for the cause. But there are few situations where the problem is not actually rooted within our psyche. Here are some examples :

1. These young women with their babies are boring: they think their children are more interesting than anyone else's. Their conversation is dull and they are ignoring me.

   Question to ask : Am I envious of their youth, and their recent motherhood?

2. The disrespect my children show me makes me angry. They have no idea what I have been through to give them what they have.

   Question to ask : Have I really done more than what any normal parent would? Do they actually wish to make me angry, and even if so, is winding me up really easy and therefore fun? No one can make me angry: I get angry on my own.

3. This job is boring and unfulfilling. The hours are too long and the pay too low.

Question to ask : How did I end up in this job? Was it a personal choice? Is it really so bad compared to other jobs? How can I change my thoughts to find this fun?

Introspection is about catching a thought in midflight and nailing it before it gets into our cells. It is a powerful tool to construct our lives around and create our days. A good strategy is to choose one of the seven deadly sins and look for signs of it during a day, or a week. For example, pride:

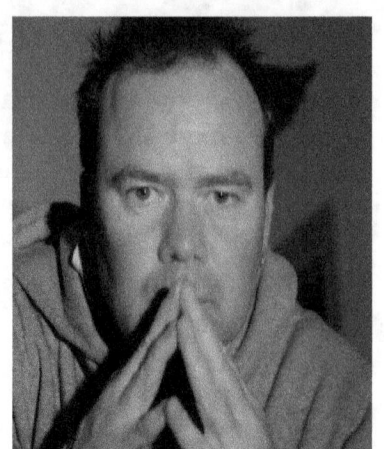

- I was so hurt by that comment. But it is my pride that it hurt. If I had more humility, the comment could not hurt me.

- I was late for a meeting because the old lady in the queue spent too long chatting to the checkout girl. I sighed and fidgeted, and my blood pressure soared. My pride told me my meeting was more important than the old lady's conversation. But in the cosmic scheme of things, maybe I am not so indispensable to the meeting, and maybe that conversation was really important to the old lady.

- I was furious when I heard about that malicious gossip about me. But if I had less pride I wouldn't be so obsessed with other people's opinion of me.

Most people live their lives in an orgy of self-justification. Introspection can lead to discovering much about ourselves we did not know and can help us subsequently eliminate thoughts, attitudes and behaviours that cause stress (DNA damage) and illness; but it also brings depth of character and understanding of others. It is an extremely powerful life tool that enriches every day when practised on a regular basis.

Man know thyself, said the inscription written on the Temple at Delphi, and thou shalt know the universe and the gods.

Setting ourselves up

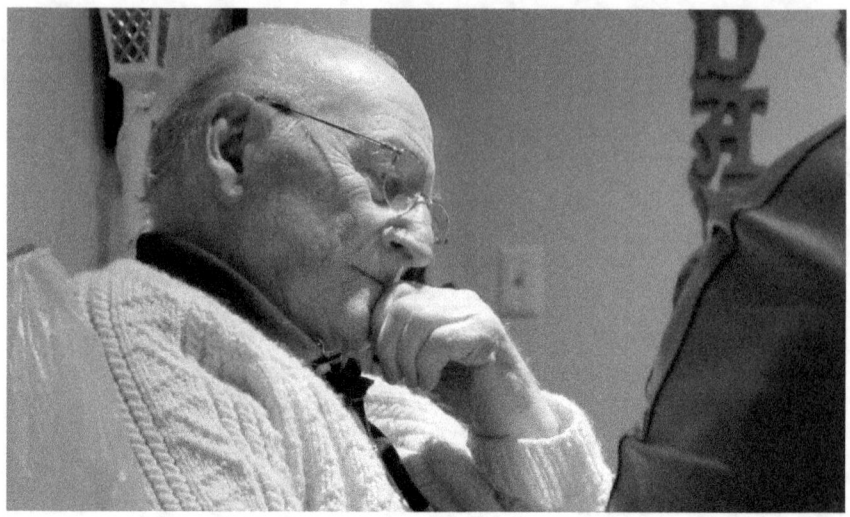

When we think about the elderly, what is the most common emotion that we feel? Studies show that pity is the first, closely followed by anxiety, probably because they remind us of what is to come. Levels of competence in older people are also estimated as being low, and research has found that when teachers were asked to give a lesson to older people, they taught less and advanced more slowly. Cognitive and physical decline is so firmly embedded in our subconscious as being an integral part of being over 65 that anyone claiming they will not decline is likely to be pitied too – because they are assumed to be in denial. There is another emotion that sometimes arises when people think of the elderly : admiration, though this is often more to do with the life they have led rather than the one they are currently leading.

In the media, older people are more likely to be shown as having some disability or as being 'difficult'. In *The Simpsons*, Homer's father is portrayed as a curmudgeon, dependent, and angry about it. Portraying seniors in negative terms – spiteful, resentful, bitter – has a subtle but strong effect on our own feelings about what we may turn out to be like in a few years. Anger at the young and at how the world has turned out, frustration at no longer being valued and stubborn adherence to outdated modes of living are stereotypes that crop up again and again. However, most of us will confirm that the 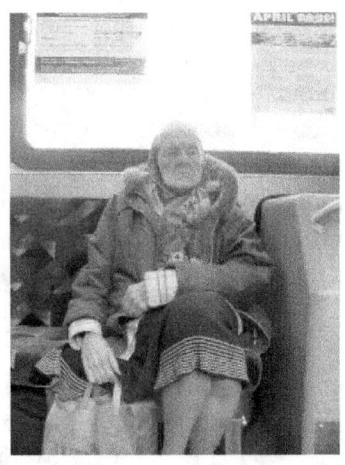 personality remains pretty much intact until death, and if someone is negative and malicious in their latter years, it is because they have been that way all their life. "If you meet a sweet little old lady," said one grandmother, "it is because she was also a sweet little young one."

Thinking of the time after retirement as one of unchecked self-indulgence and regret is setting ourselves up. Even if we prefer the image of the wise old-timer or peaceful older woman giving sound advice, this too is a form of marginalisation. Equating seniority with the end of a spiritual journey detracts from the physical and removes older people from active life; it holds older adults to a different standard than the one we are setting for everyone else, and remaining young, vibrant and active can be seen as depriving ourselves of the wisdom that comes with age.

Older people themselves are vulnerable to negative age-related stereotypes. One study (Hess, Hinson & Hodges 2009) had older participants take a memory test. One group was told the test was to assess the impact of ageing on memory and the other group was not informed that age was a factor. The first group did worse, and the highly educated in the 'informed' group did worst of all.

The eclipse of our mental powers fills those of us who have used them to the full all our lives with such a sense of dread that we may end up with a spiraling form of ageism, where anxiety about getting old, plus our own prejudices about our elders, can lead to underperformance and a self-fulfilling prophecy. The risk of internalising the 'old fool' stereotype is particularly acute. Self-identifying as being old is also far more threatening than identifying with some other vulnerable group, since ethnic minorities, homosexuals or the disabled for example have had a lifetime to adjust to membership, whereas it is the abrupt threshold of retirement age that foists senior citizenship upon us. Suddenly we find we are members of a new club we never wanted to join, and have to cope with all the stereotypes we had in our own minds about that club when we were young. Refusing to join in may be seen as arrogant, isolationist or even downright antisocial. Accepting old age 'graciously' is often code for giving up part of ourselves.

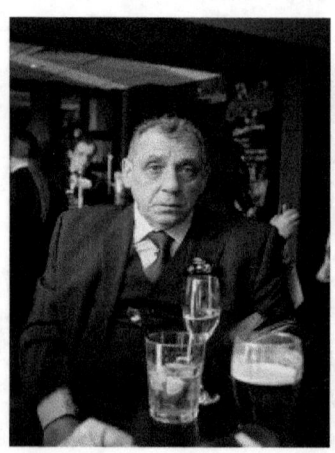

In the collective unconscious older people seem to fall into two categories – wise and removed from the turmoil of life, or ill and suffering from the terrible burdens of old age such that death is preferable. Paying in advance for a place in an assisted living home is the best way of ensuring we will one day require it. Treating the elderly as somehow different from everyone else is setting ourselves up for marginalisation in later life.

In making assumptions of those who were born before us we are preparing the way for ourselves later on.

The Superstar Butcher

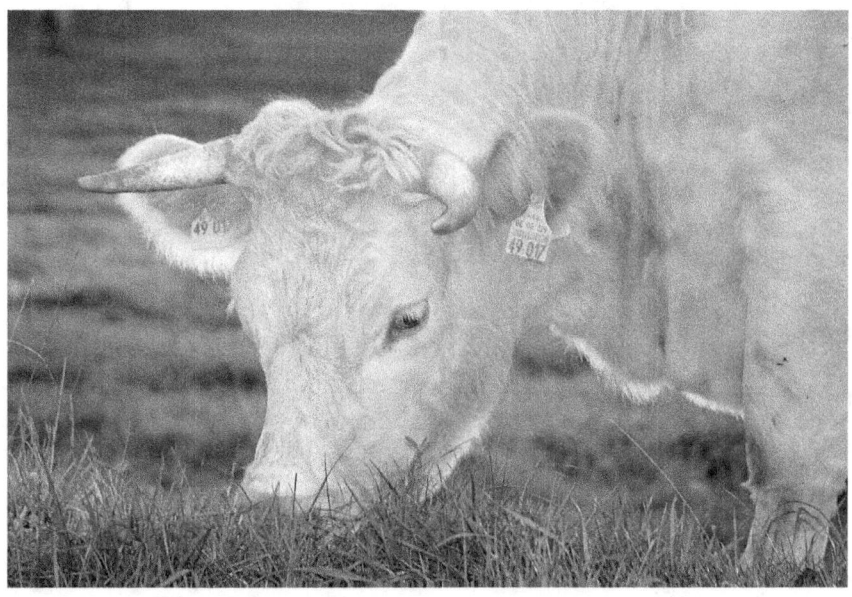

Hugo Desnoyer is France's most famous butcher, supplier to the stars and the best restaurants in Paris. Queues form outside his shop every morning, and customers regularly spend thousands of euros on his top quality meat. He is known for having transformed the image of butcher from ruffian to superstar, rehabilitating the coarse tradesman with a blood-stained apron brandishing a knife into a connoisseur and advisor to France's elite. He is famed as an author and expert in the ingredients of haute cuisine, and as a keen promoter of animal welfare.

Desnoyer selects and regularly visits the farms which rear his animals and the abattoirs where they are slaughtered. People buy his meat because he ensures the animals are played classical music to relax them in the moments preceding slaughter. It is the reason

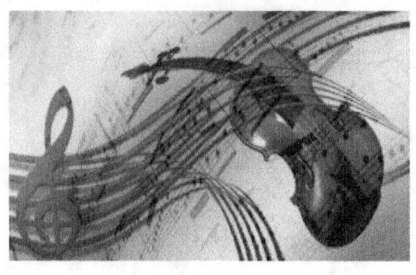

for this measure that is so intriguing. He claims that the meat tastes completely different if the animal was anxious or experiencing distress before its death, saying, "The animals must never be under stress. If they are, the meat will be full of knots and saturated with an acidic taste. Even the best quality animal will produce nothing worth eating if it is under stress."

Studies around the world have proven that music reduces stress in animals. It not only improves meat quality, it increases milk yield in cows, and on some farms in Italy buffalos listen to Mozart three times a day to help them produce better mozzarella milk. Playing classical music in tube stations and in tough areas reduces crime. It helps premature babies thrive and reduces road rage to such an extent that the German transport minister issued an *Adagio in the Automobile* CD to reduce aggressive driving on the country's autobahns.

What has this got to do with staying ageless?

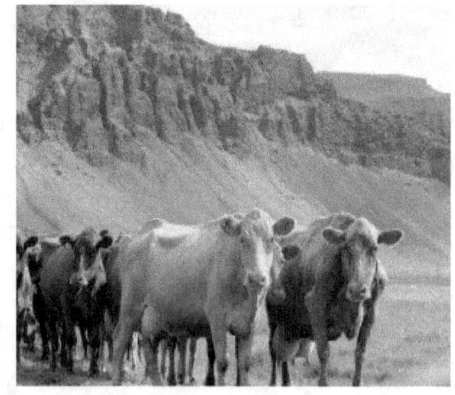

The message from farming is clear : what stress does to animals, it also does to us. Stress management techniques, both in our external actions and in directing our thoughts, are crucial in promoting and maintaining health.

I Can't Sleep

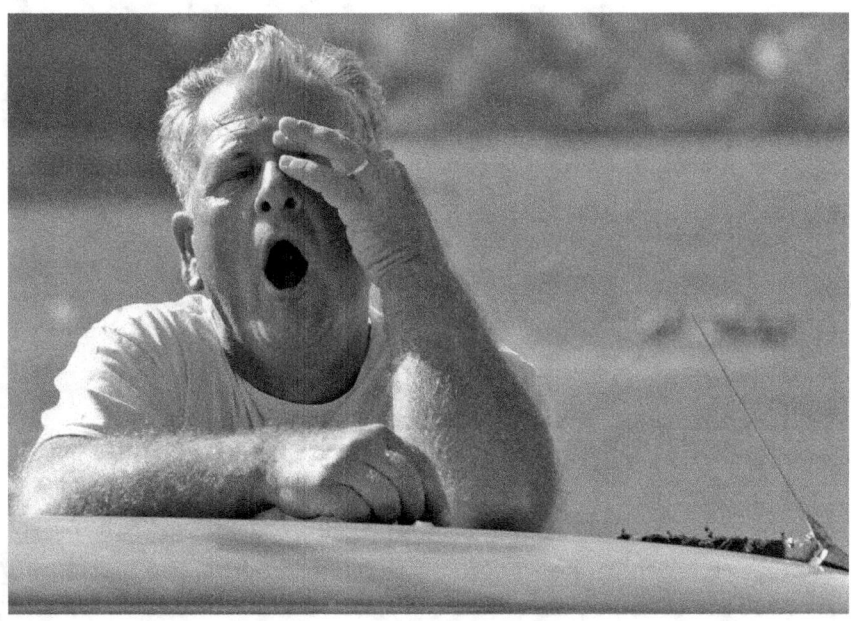

You spent your entire working life dreaming for the days when you can have a lie-in every day, and when they come you find you can't sleep later than 7am. Crazy or what? As the years pass, our sleep patterns change. Our circadian rhythms are reset, and earlier nights and earlier mornings become more normal. The transition between being asleep and awake is more sudden, making us feel we are now light sleepers, and lower levels of growth hormone restrict deep sleep; we may find ourselves waking up more often during the night, sometimes to go to the toilet. We may want to take naps during the day.

However, feeling tired all the time is not normal at any age. Sleep is vital to allow the body to repair cell damage that occurred during the day. It strengthens the immune system which in turn reduces the risk of disease. Not getting a good night's sleep can be a factor in cancer, sleep apnea (breathing problems), cardiovascular disease, diabetes and obesity. Worse, it can lead to concentration problems (at any age), and impaired neurocognition. And then when we rise, we look like we've been in a natural disaster. Sleep problems also cause skin ageing – less moisture, more fine lines, uneven texture and slackening according to a study commissioned by Estee Lauder.

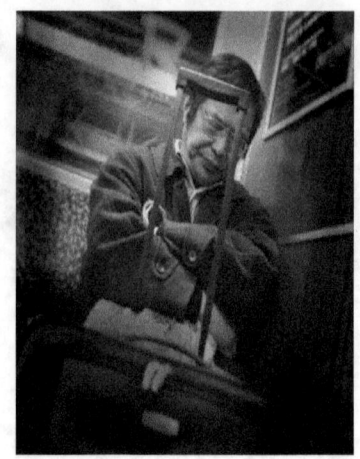

So what if we can't sleep? If we work in bed, then the mind does not associate bed with just sleeping, and that's one area we can control. So no i-pads, or TV. Daily exercise, no stimulants in the evening and pain relief help, as does journalling or talking to someone about things that we are worried about. Earplugs can help us cope with the freight-train snorer in our lives and a bedtime ritual such as soft music or sounding a Tibetan bowl as we lie down can also trigger the sleep response.

If we find we can't get to sleep, two things always help :

• Don't look at the clock. Calculating how long it has been since we went to bed and how many hours there are left before we have to get up again will make things worse the next day, since our minds will tell us, "I only got x hours sleep". Ignorance is bliss during the small hours.

• Say, "Although I am not sleeping, I am resting my mind and my body. This is good, and almost the same thing."

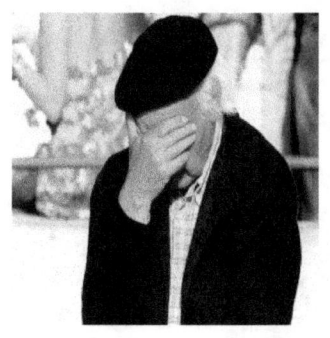

The most ageing thing about not sleeping is worrying we are not sleeping. Not the lack of sleep.

Seven Ways to Change Your DNA

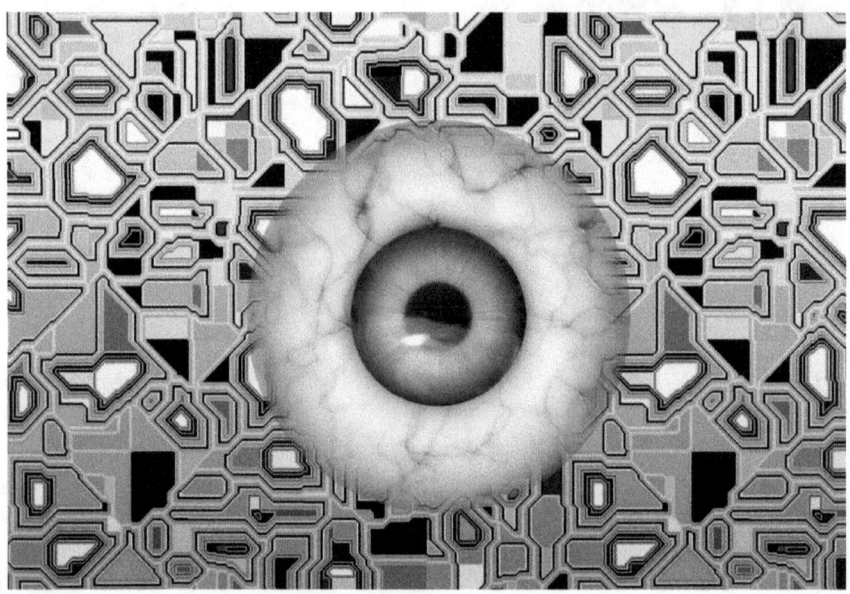

Is there anyone left who still believes in genetic determinism?

It is now accepted that DNA is not our destiny. While anyone claiming you can change your DNA would have been laughed out of the room a few years ago, once again science fiction has turned out to be fact, and the science of epigenetics shows that more than anything the environment – inner and outer – determines our health and longevity.

Obviously we are all born with a DNA sequence. Our general appearance is dictated at birth. However lifestyle, our emotional world and what happens to us greatly affect how we look. These external factors to our DNA switch genes on and off all the time. The science of switching on genes is known as epigenetics.

Since the discovery of genes a creeping victim mentality has overtaken the world. If we can do nothing about our genetic heritage then why bother trying to live longer and more healthily? Genetic determinism created a culture of irresponsibility and recklessness about our health. When your time's up, your time's up went the saying.

Not so fast. Even if a disease runs in a family, and even if we have inherited the gene for it, through lifestyle and mindfulness there is a huge amount we can do to prevent triggering that gene. Research (at the University of Bologna) is beginning to show that DNA can be altered through magnetic fields, positive mental states and – crucially though this is still controversial – intention. Since all cells contain the same DNA, but differentiate to form skin, organs or bone for example, research is being done to reprogramme cells back to a state where they can redifferentiate into any cell in the body. So far it has been shown we can change our DNA expression in the following ways:

• Meditation. The relaxation response was studied in groups of individuals in the US, France and Spain. After just eight hours of meditation, the individuals showed molecular differences, altered levels of gene-regulation and reduced levels of pro-inflammatory genes, which promotes rapid recovery from stress. "To the best of our knowledge, this is the first paper that shows rapid alterations in gene expression associated with mindfulness meditation practice," says study author Richard J. Davidson, founder of the Center for Investigating Healthy Minds and the William James and Vilas Professor of Psychology and Psychiatry at the University of Wisconsin-Madison. "Most interestingly, the changes were observed in genes that are the current targets of anti-inflammatory and analgesic drugs," says Perla Kaliman, a researcher at the

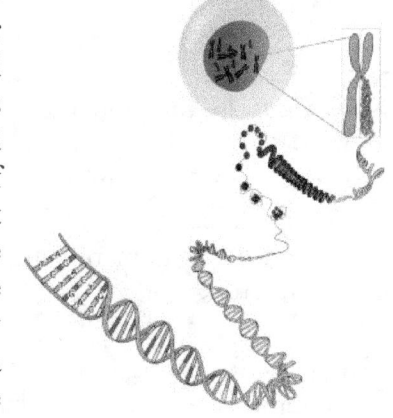

Institute of Biomedical Research of Barcelona, Spain where the molecular analyses were conducted.

• Therapy and changing learned behaviour. Eric Kandel the Austrian-American neuropsychiatrist and Nobel Prize winner has claimed that psychotherapy produces changes in gene expression that alter the anatomical pattern of nerve cells in the brain.

• Stress reduction techniques (leisure activities, changing negative thoughts etc...) These 'psychosocial' techniques are thought to change gene expression and alter brain structure.

• Intentionality. At the Institute of HeartMath in Boulder Creek, an experienced meditator was given three DNA samples and was instructed to unwind two through intentional visualisation. By creating a calm state of emotional and physical harmony the meditator succeeded in unwinding two samples and left the third unchanged. If further experiments confirm that this is possible, then DNA visualisation techniques in meditation are a powerful way of controlling our ageing and our health.

• Exercise. Researchers compared activity in muscle-related genes before and after exercise. After a single 20 minute workout the participants' DNA showed less methylation (a molecular process involved in ageing). Methylation is a process in which chemicals called methyl groups land on the DNA and limit the cells' ability to access, or switch on, certain genes.

• Beliefs. Eric Kandel concluded that many genetic differences between us are due to conditioning and the society we grew up in, rather than fixed in the raw material we inherited from our parents. However, there is growing evidence that these epigenetic changes can be included in the DNA passed on to the next generation, a theory known as Lamarckism which until recently was discredited as an old wives' tale.

• Diet. The following foods reduce DNA methylation:
- cruciferous vegetables, e.g. broccoli, cauliflower.
- foods high in folic acid, e.g. liver, egg yolk, dried beans.

- foods high in antioxidants, e.g. berries.
- foods high in vitamin B12, e.g. liver, meat, eggs.
- foods high in amino acids and B complex vitamins, e.g. spinach, eggs.

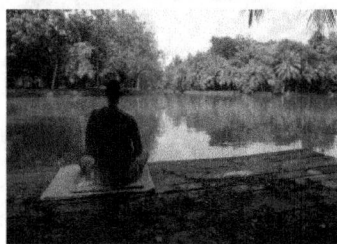 99.9% of our genes are the same. The differences between us depend on which genes are switched on. This in turn depends on the environment and social conditioning of certain beliefs and behaviours.

So, good news again. We can control our destiny

Music – a quick fix

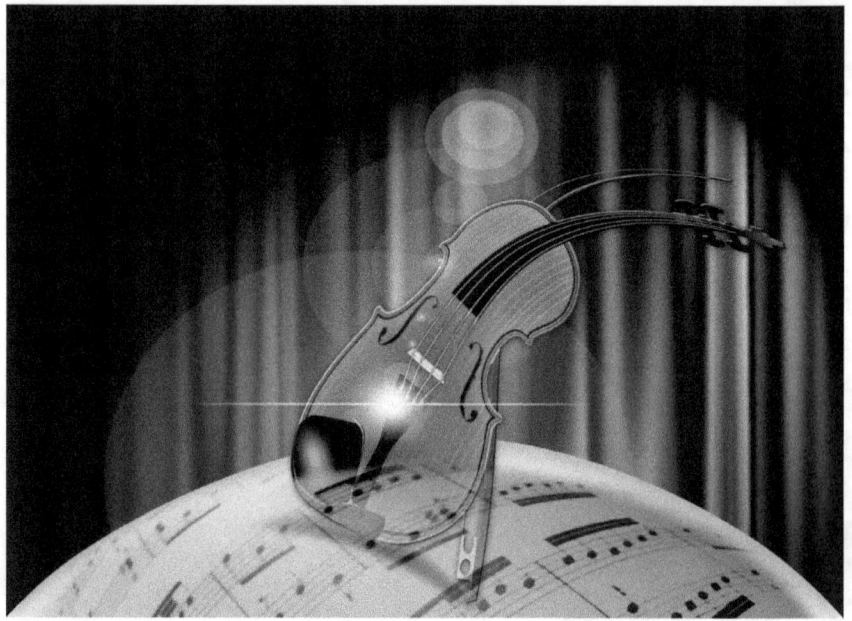

Stress is turning out to be the number one factor in ageing. Neither healthy food, nor exercise, nor pills can counteract the body's stress response if stress is persistent, but one way of combatting stress which is free and readily available is music.

Music increases immunoglobulin A and natural killer cell counts in our blood, protecting us from infection. It is the fastest and most efficient way of changing mood, with almost immediate effect – far faster than talking therapy (and cheaper). It reduces the secretion of stress hormones which have such a devastating impact on telomere length. Listening to music boosts dopamine and causes the cerebral cortex to produce either alpha waves for relaxation or beta waves (lively music) if we need energy. These days nothing is true until a lab has verified it, but countless scientific studies have shown the positive effects on health of music. These include :

• Normalisation of heart beat, blood pressure and blood vessel function (crucial when we are stressed) and reduction of anxiety.

• Speeding up recovery from stroke – music works faster than listening to stories in helping patients to regain verbal skills and body coordination.

• Releasing endorphins to reduce pain.

• Boosting memory and concentration, particularly baroque music with its 60 beats per minute, by stimulating both the left and right brain.

• Improving sleep patterns.

• Relieving depression – avoiding sad music or music that enhances bad memories but instead choosing music which does not match our depressed mood. We may feel the music jars with our state, but this is a leap of faith that works.

• Combatting anger. Listening to music in the car reduces irritation and road rage.

• Enhancing exercise performance. Music can reduce the impression of effort, and upbeat music has been shown to boost the performance of professional sportsmen and women.

• Soothing and regulating our cells and vital organs.

Music distracts us from a bad situation. It changes our mood and alters our thoughts. It nudges us towards a better state of

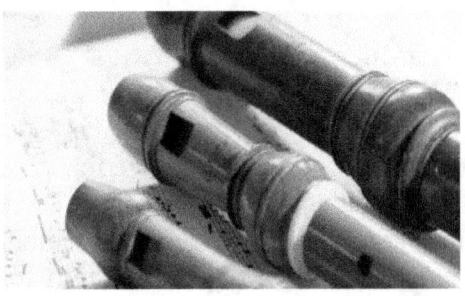

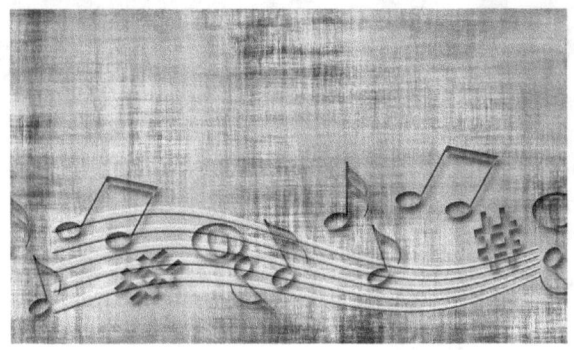 mind. Becoming absorbed in a piece of music we enjoy has the strange effect of giving us back a sense of control when we feel we are losing it.

If we cannot meditate, or have a massage, music is an easy emergency stop option that can stop us sinking into the kind of rumination which makes us grow old before our time.

Here are two Baroque pieces which have an immediate effect on mood:

Tomaso Albinoni : Concerto Op.5 No. 7 in D minor

When we are worried about something this piece seems to recognise our state of anxiety while placing it in a wider perspective. The melody changes back and forth from minor to major and ends in a triumphant tone. After listening to the piece in a meditative state this music uplifts and makes worries seem less important. This concerto brings closure. We live in a big world.

Antonio Vivaldi : Concerto No. 4 in F minor ('Winter' from the Four Seasons)

This piece boosts self-esteem, raises hopefulness and puts trials and hardship in perspective. It is good for those who feel wronged, those hesitating over a decision, who need to find energy to carry out a task or take an important step in personal development. Above all, it provides an injection of self-confidence and optimism while recognising the instinct to tread carefully at first. It is at times quite an angry piece, and demonstrates how intense irritation or even feelings of rage can be transformed into the energy needed to change things. The finale reminds the listener there is always an amazing surprise around the corner, reaching a crescendo of personal energy and resolve.

Photo Credit: _zhang via Compfight cc

Subatomic meditation

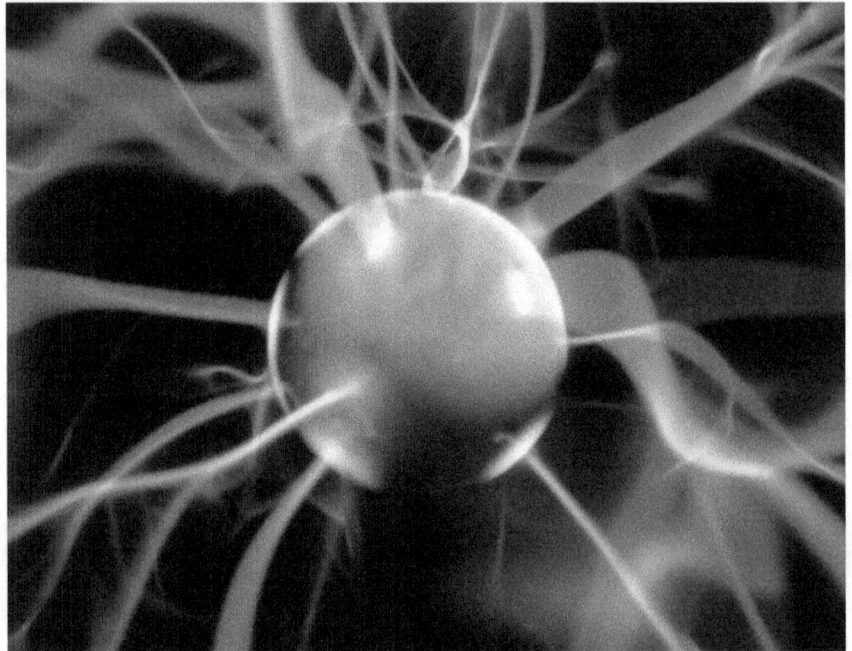

Here is a meditation that descends deep into the cell at the subatomic level.

We imagine we are standing outside a cell in our body. This may be a symbol for all our body or the cell of a particular area we wish to heal or rejuvenate. We see the cell wall, penetrate through a receptor crossing the cytoplasm to the nucleus. With an attitude of reverence we penetrate the nucleus where we encounter chromosomes made up of the triple helix – DNA. We become even smaller and see that the triple helix is made up of a chain of molecules (carbon, nitrogen, hydrogen, oxygen..), and that each DNA molecule is made up of atoms. We picture these atoms, and choose one. Then we enter the atom, the smallest unit of life. We are on holy ground.

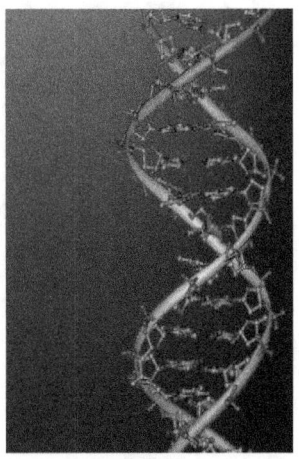

Our consciousness has now entered the subatomic level. At this level time is fuzzy and electrons can be in several places at once. The subatomic particles that exist in our bodies can exist as a wave or as a particle.

Picture then, the interior of an atom inside our bodies. The atom is made up of a nucleus of neutrons and protons, bunched together like grapes, and electrons in orbit in what is known as electron shells around the nucleus.

In a flash we find ourselves sitting on top of the nucleus, and we behold the sky above us. The electrons are in a cloud, and can only be seen if we fix our attention on them, otherwise the sensation is that we are surrounded by a crackling fog. Here and there like forked lightning are the electron trails which slowly fade away like vapour. In the first orbit two electrons can be made out if we fix our focus there. In the second – further out – there are eight, in the third eighteen...

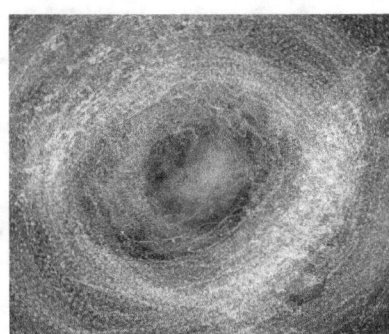

We see ourselves then, on the surface of the nucleus, looking up at the cloud of electrons that appear and disappear from behind the clouds like moons in orbit around a strange planet. We visualise the lights, the colours of the electron cloud above.

The distances are vast – the electron shells extend as far as the eye can see. This is the subatomic field. We have placed our focus in the enormous empty space that makes up 99.99% of our bodies. We are, at this moment in our meditation, pure consciousness with power over the matter beneath us. And so we repeat:

"Regeneration is more natural than degeneration."

When we wish to end our meditation, we rise up through the electron cloud and exit the atom, the nucleus and the cell, and open our eyes, gazing upwards imagining the sun and the moon above us and the endless spaces beyond.

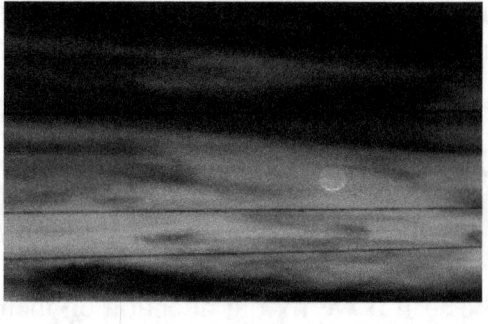

When depression comes BEFORE the thoughts

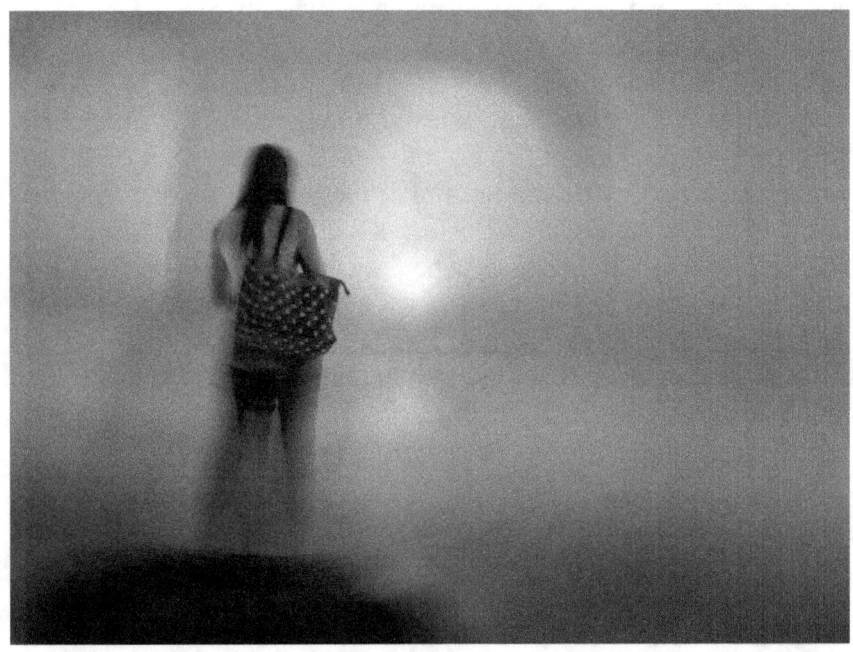

Ever felt really depressed and couldn't work out why?

The problem arises when we wake up, feel depressed, and then our mind seeks a reason to justify the depression. There are always reasons in our life to be depressed. Even if everything is going well, we may fear losing the happy state, or feel guilt over having achieved something others didn't, or about an argument with someone recently. We feel something is bound to go wrong if it hasn't already, and the downward spiral begins. Taking antidepressants may correct the chemical issue in the short term, but it fails to address the root cause. Pinpointing the original thought or emotion that is niggling us is the first step towards changing our mental state. Sometimes these emotions can be traced back to something someone said days or even weeks ago.

Rumination is now being shown to be one of the key causes of ageing and illness. If we fail to recognise wallowing for the health compromiser that it is, we are playing Russian roulette with our bodies. We must recognise that our thoughts are profoundly influenced by our mood, and that when we are depressed, this is not who we really are. Sad, defeatist thoughts are alien invaders, which we must wipe out if we value our health. In times of despair when we are too raw even to think, repetitive chants can sooth us into a gentler mental state. Countless studies have confirmed that chanting reverses depression. Chanting has been shown to block the release of stress hormones, normalise adrenalin and lower cholesterol, as well as filling the mind so it cannot focus on sad and depressing ideas. It is therefore not hocus-pocus but a tried and tested remedy against ill health. There are many different chants but one easy one is *Om shanti shanti shanti.*

Depression is harmful to our health, and speeds up ageing. It can lead to weight gain, heart disease, insomnia, and aches and pains. Low levels of serotonin can lower our pain threshold, and stress hormones make us more susceptible to disease. Health problems associated with depression include diabetes, stroke, digestive issues, cancer, kidney disease, arthritis and autoimmune conditions

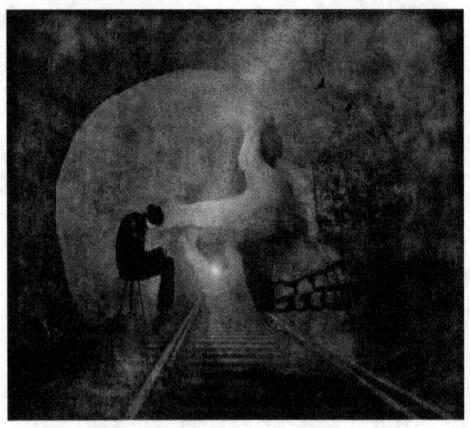

such as lupus and Parkinson's. Depression may start in the head, but the effects on the body are soon felt if it is not addressed. If we are tempted to wallow, the spectre of physical problems to add to our emotional ones should spur us on to change our mental landscape.

Sometimes an underlying medical disorder can trigger a chemical imbalance which leads to depression, but as depression also triggers chemical imbalances….well, could be chicken and egg.

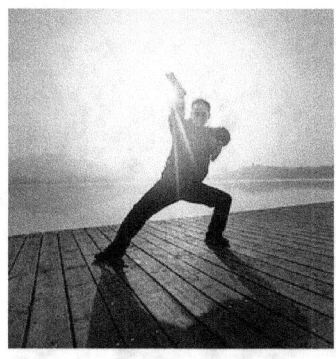

Morning depression is sometimes a hangover from sleep; it can also be due to Seasonal Affected Disorder, thought to be caused by the hibernation response left over from our biological ancestors. Lack of serotonin may play a role in SAD, but however little we feel like it, the symptoms can soon be overcome by engaging in physical activity or exposing ourselves to light.

Even if the cause of depression is hormonal, such as in premenstrual syndrome, MRI scans have now proven beyond doubt that changes in our thinking can change brain chemistry. This is a fantastic piece of news that gives us mastery over not only our lives but our bodies too.

Telomeres – the long and the short of it.

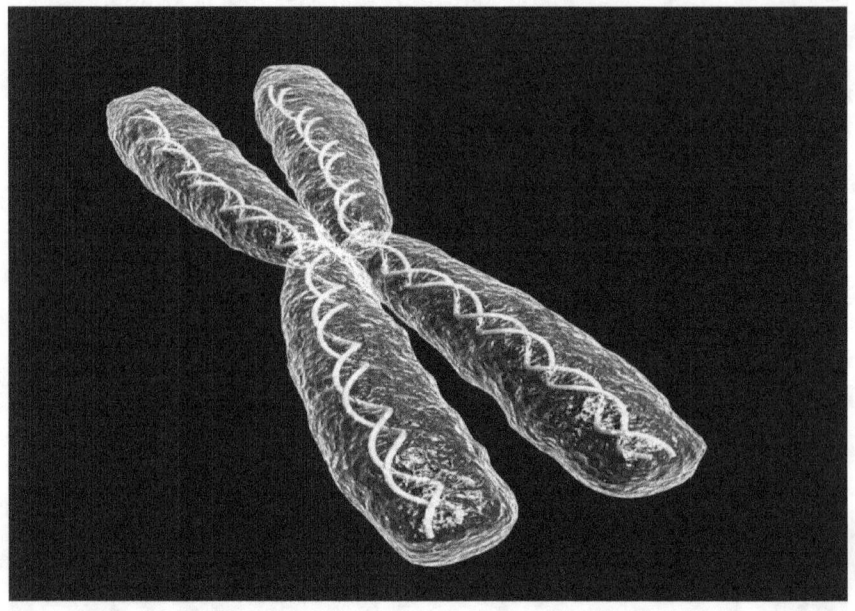

In September 2013 one of the most empowering research outcomes ever was published in *The Lancet Oncology*. It concerned telomeres, the strands at the end of our chromosomes. The research, according to lead author Dean Ornish, UCSF clinical professor of medicine, concluded that genes are not necessarily our fate. The study focused on a group of men with early-stage prostate cancer. Half of the group were instructed to continue as normal; the other half made lifestyle changes. These changes involved a low-fat, plant-based diet, low in refined carbs, moderate exercise (walking for half an hour a day), yoga or meditation for an hour a day (to combat stress) and spending more time with friends and loved ones.

At the end of the five year study their telomeres were measured, and it was found that in the group which had changed their lifestyle, their telomeres had lengthened by ten percent. Men in the other group had a 3 percent shortening of telomeres over this period.

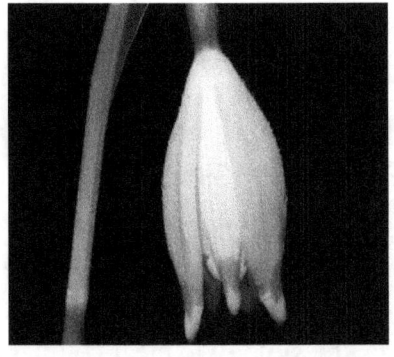

Why is this amazing news?

Scientists have been fascinated by telomeres since they were discovered to hold the key to our biological age. It was found that the older we get, the shorter our telomeres are, and the shorter our telomeres, the shorter our lives. It had been conceded that the shortening of telomeres was, however, not entirely dependent on genes, but that hardship and stress accelerated the rate at which they shrank. Factors contributing to early telomere shortening were thought to be smoking, radiation exposure, taking care of relatives with Alzheimer's or autistic children as well as regular exposure to emotional stress such a bad marriage or high pressure at work. The study measured telomeres in white blood cells, not in the prostate, making it relevant to the entire population. Although this was only a small pilot study it is significant; most research begins with small studies such as this one. It showed that the more lifestyle changes were made, the longer the telomeres got.

It appears our cells are listening to our suffering. Until now the possibility of lengthening telomeres was seen as something only possible in science fiction, akin to actual rejuvenation, an attitude very much in line with the widespread belief ageing is inevitable, still so prevalent today.

Telomeres then are not age-dependent, in fact it has been found that centenarians have longer telomeres than most 85-year-olds, and it is thought that it is not the telomeres that have given them long life, but that their long lives are attributable to better health, which was reflected in the telomeres. Clearly changes in lifestyle affect cellular ageing.

Cancer cells also have longer telomeres, and this is one of the main reasons attempts to produce an elixir of life based on telomerase for example face so many difficulties. Cancer cells produce telomerase. Aubrey de Grey of the SENS foundation which studies rejuvenation said, "The cancer problem is a really, really big problem."

This study however indicates that high tech drugs are probably not the answer. Instead low-tech non-medical intervention seems to be extremely effective. Our bodies have a remarkable capacity to heal themselves. Being a victim of abuse, suffering emotionally, allowing negative emotions to dictate our lives and enduring hardship are not irreversible blows to the body. If we make the changes now, using techniques such as kinesiology to clear cellular memory, recognising and combatting stress whenever it appears and practising calorie restriction to reduce oxidative damage, then we can take back control of the ageing process and – as the telomere study seems to suggest – reverse it.

The Philosopher's Stone

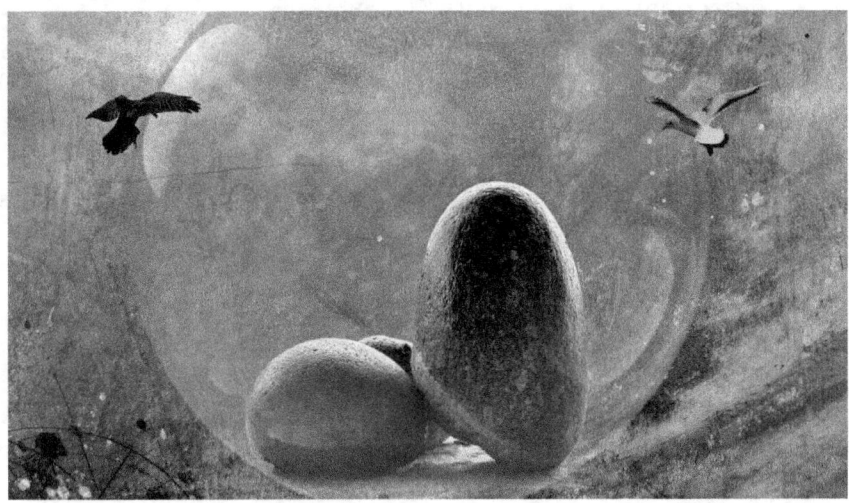

Sir Isaac Newton's alchemical papers were only rediscovered in the middle of the twentieth century, and they revealed that Newton was an alchemist first and a physicist second. Though not generally known as an alchemist, he was fascinated by the art. In fact it has been claimed that it was the inspiration for his theory of light and gravity. He wrote over a million words on the subject, but the Royal Society refused to print them after his death. The Newtonian worldview, where science and mechanics rule the universe, turns out to be not Newtonian at all, since Sir Isaac was deeply interested in spiritual, indeed occult matters. John Maynard Keynes the economist famously said of him, "He was not the first of the age of reason, but the last of the magicians." Several documents indicate Newton's interest in finding the Philosopher's Stone, believed to be the source of the Elixir of Life, a means of achieving rejuvenation and even immortality. On an external, worldly level it was described as a substance capable of turning base metals into gold, but the spiritual meaning of the Stone, which is of course a metaphor, is enlightenment.

It is a universal symbol :
mention of it can be found in
ancient Greek writings
(Zosimos of Panopolis) and
in Hindu scriptures where it
is known as the Cintamani
and is depicted as a fabulous
jewel. It is Western
mysticism's symbol for
sexual magic – the phallic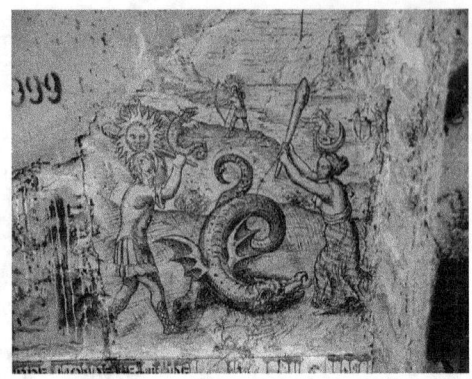
symbol of the Sword in the Stone legend, which confers kingship
on those who pursue the goal of rejuvenation and immortality,
mirroring the promises of Eastern tantra. Excalibur conferred
supernatural powers on the bearer; the wounds inflicted by
Excalibur would draw no blood. In his work "Atalanta Fugiens",
the German physician and alchemist Michael Maier says : "Make
of a man and woman a circle; then a quadrangle; out of this a
triangle; make again a circle, and you will have the Stone of the
Wise. Thus is made the stone, which thou canst not discover,
unless you, through diligence, learn to understand this geometrical
teaching." The "geometrical teaching" is clearly connected to the
combination of male and female energies. The Philosopher's Stone
is a metaphor for immortality, just as the stone altar in a church
symbolises the sacred spot where the priest unites the divine and
the material. Jesus said to Peter, "on this rock I will build my
church" in response to his statement that Jesus is the embodiment
of the unity of the divine and the earthly. It is used as a metaphor
again in the Book of Peter, which urges believers to be living
stones, and some mystics have interpreted Exodus 17 as a veiled
tantric symbol; Moses uses his staff to touch the rock, and out
flows fresh water for the thirsty Israelites in the desert.

Alchemy is not really about physical lead and gold, but is a natural
art available to all those who have an open mind about their own
power to bring healing and long life to themselves. Various sources
describe the Philosopher's Stone as a common substance, to be
found everywhere, but which is normally unrecognised. The
Philosopher's Stone is not made by the alchemist; it is there
already in Nature waiting to be discovered. The alchemist simply

provides the physical conditions – within his or her own body, through channeling of sexual energy and transformation of negative thoughts and lower passions – to allow Nature to work without hindrance from the misconceptions of the mind. It means, to be clear, man taking control of his life, converting the base metal of his mind and body to the gold of spiritual enlightenment. It is about the combination of creative and healing forces, balancing the feminine and masculine aspects of the spirit to create what the alchemists called the sacred hermaphrodite from the fires of human passion.

The Philosopher's Stone is the symbol of man's eternal dream to find a way to overcome disease and death, and to finally take control.

Can We Rebuild Ourselves?

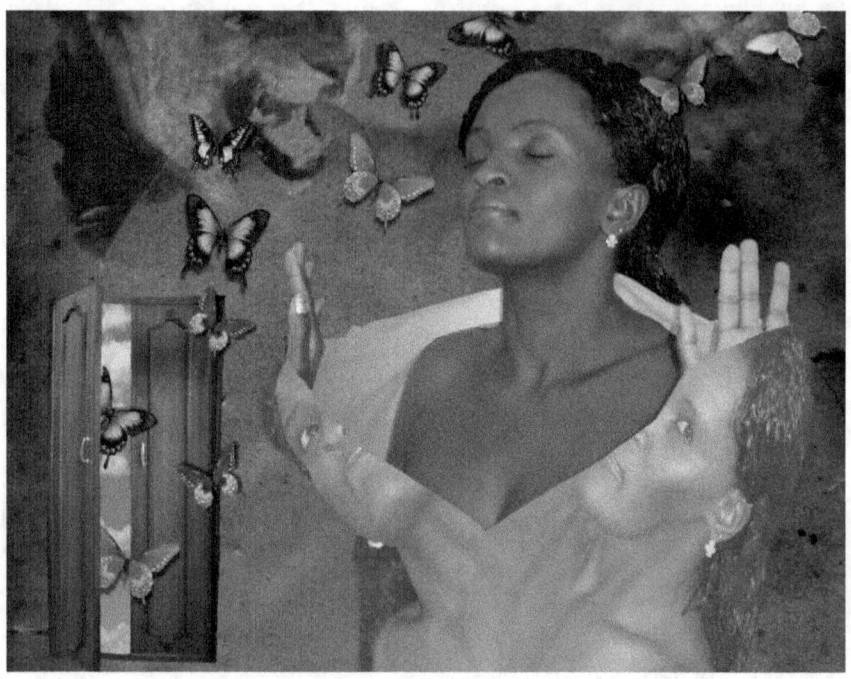

In the 1970s hit television series *The Six Million Dollar Man*, when astronaut Steve Austin is severely injured in a crash, his body is rebuilt using bionic implants. Imagine for a moment that whenever our body was damaged, however seriously, we could regenerate the organ or limb until they were as good as new. Of course in nature this is nothing out of the ordinary. In fact every species, including humans, is capable of regeneration. Human foetuses can regrow everything from hearts to limbs if they are damaged in the womb, and in adults nails, hair, bones and skin all regenerate. The adult liver is one of the most regenerative organs and can rebuild itself from only one quarter of the original mass. Amphibians and reptiles can also regenerate legs, tails, jaws, eyes and a variety of internal structures. They do this by rearranging existing tissue or

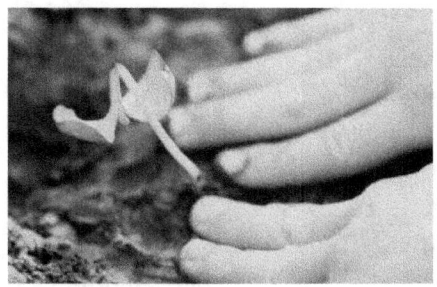

by the differentiation of adult cells into stem cells, which then develop into new tissue the same way the part developed in the first place.

Scientists are reviewing their opinion that regenerating lost or damaged tissue is the stuff of science fiction. Studies have shown that children up to the age of 10 who lose fingertips in accidents can regrow the tip within a month, provided that their wounds are not sealed up with flaps of skin – the standard treatment. The new digit normally won't have a fingerprint, and if there is any piece of the fingernail left it will grow back too, though in a square rather than oval shape.

The use of an extract from pig's bladder called 'extracellular matrix' has shown that adults can also regrow fingers. Extracellular matrix acts as a sort of scaffolding for cells to regrow on. It organises the signals that direct cells to form a certain shape. It is made up of collagen, and does not contain any cells as such (so there is no chance amputees might regrow a trotter). Usually scar tissue forms over a wound, to prevent any cellular development in the area, which is why scars are permanent – no cells can move in to do a repair job. This is as a result of the immune system trying to prevent the dead cells around the wound seeping into the surrounding tissue. When extracellular matrix is applied to a wound, it instead causes the cells to start repairing the damage rather than creating scar tissue.

In 2005 Lee Spievack accidently sliced off the tip of his right middle finger. By chance his brother Dr Alan Spievack was researching regeneration and covered the wound with powdered extracellular matrix developed by Dr Stephen Badylak of the McGowan Institute of Regenerative Medicine. The missing fingertip regrew in four weeks. In a similar case a woman named Deepa Kulkarni lost the tip of her little finger. She refused to believe doctors that nothing could be done, and thanks to Dr Badylak's regenerative therapy her little finger grew back. The question is, if our extracellular matrix stops working after birth, how can humans trigger it to start working again? Experiments on mice have already succeeded in preventing extracellular matrix from being switched off by manipulating the gene responsible (Lin28a), leading to the mice being able to repair and heal wounds which would otherwise have been permanent. Extracellular matrix is currently being tested on Iraq War veterans whose hands were damaged in the war, by reopening the wounds and applying the matrix to the stubs. Even if the entire fingers do not grow back, the hope is that enough of the fingers will reappear to allow them to be usable.

It is clear that we are at the beginnings of bringing science fiction into the realms of fact. There are 10 million amputees worldwide. Regrowing an entire limb may seem an impossibility, but it is not. Nature does it already : deer antlers – regenerated every year – are made up of cartilage, bone and skin just like legs are. This has implications for the replacement of ageing organs and for the regeneration of eyes, ears, hearts and lungs – and in the beauty industry, the regeneration of ageing skin and muscle.

Dental Hygiene and Ageing

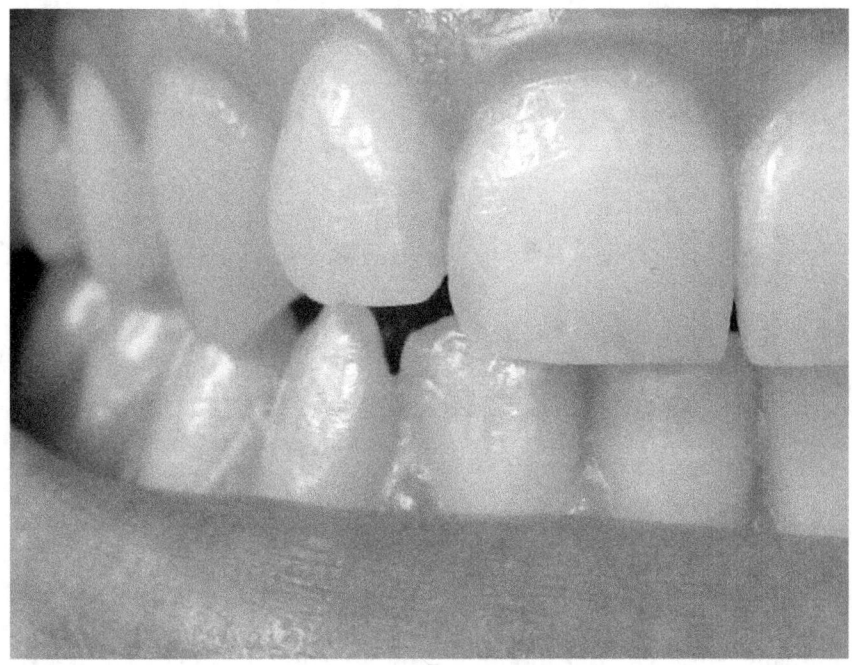

"You have a choice," said the dentist with a big, white smile. "Either you go for implants or your face will slowly collapse, your jaw will jut forward Neanderthal-style and you will never eat steak again." The patient reached deep into her pocket, and chose the implants.

The spectre of the chomping older person who has forgotten to put their teeth in is a social archetype many of us grew up with, but dentistry has advanced since then, and having one's dentures in a glass as a night companion is no longer our inevitable fate. However, worn, grey or crooked teeth can add years to our appearance – no wonder that for centuries horse traders looked at an animal's teeth to judge its age. While most people over 65 still have some of their natural teeth, they unsurprisingly suffer from more decay, gum disease and mouth infections than any other group. Receding gums, wobbly teeth and deterioration of the jaw bone make matters worse, and bacteria from poor dental hygiene affect the rest of our bodies, having been linked to diabetes, stroke, respiratory disease and heart attacks.

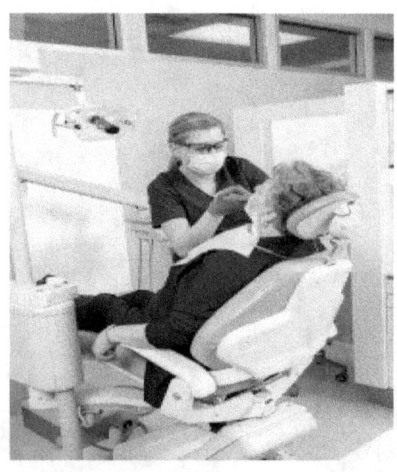

Stress often leads to teeth grinding and often we aren't even aware we are doing it; a lot of pressure will be placed on the back teeth which can cause jaw pain, ear ache and increased tooth sensitivity. If we haven't flossed before, now is the time to start adding it to our twice-daily brushing regime, preferably with an electric toothbrush, with the use of mouthwash to disinfect. If the teeth are too far gone, implants can give your mouth a truly amazing new lease of life, so they are well worth the investment. Veneers will bring back that Hollywood smile, though they involve grinding down the original teeth and placing porcelain jackets over them. For a less radical solution we can regularly whiten our teeth using the many methods available through dentists and chemists, including wearing gum shield-like trays at night containing a bleaching agent or laser treatment which activates the chemicals, though not everyone gets teeth the colour of snow. Conclusion : protecting our mouths from ageing will protect the rest of us too.

Remembering the Future

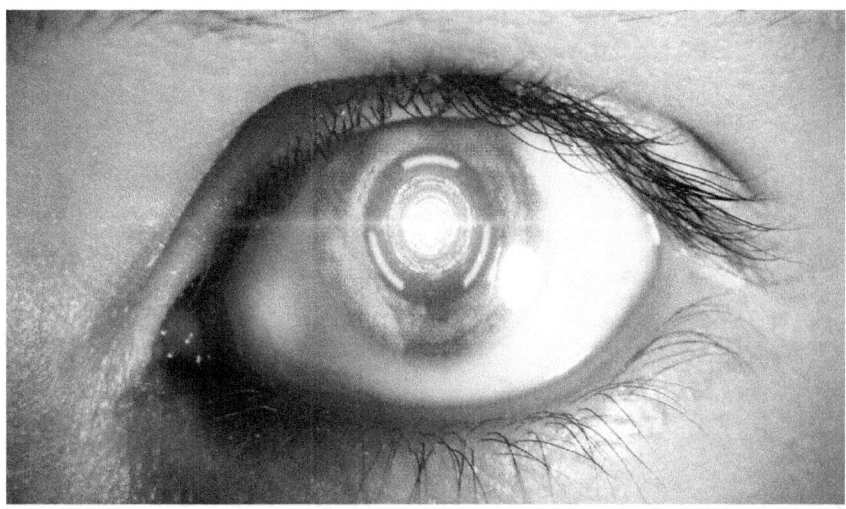

Have we ever brought ourselves to tears thinking about something which never happened?

Our past experiences and things we have learnt have set up entire networks of electrons in the brain. However, when we start to speculate, or imagine something in the future, researchers are beginning to show the brain can also remember the future. Every time we visualise a future outcome the network is strengthened. The brain can dip into different networks based on past information and emotions and create a new network which forms an image. Eventually the brain is structured as if the event has already occurred, and the body receives messages from this circuitry. So thinking about and feeling what a future experience may look like will affect your personal reality now. The body is getting the signal before the event has occurred, and it does not know the difference.

Consciousness remains a mystery. Some scientists believe it is a biological phenomenon, different from mental and physical processes but somehow concurrent with life and a property of the brain. Others have suggested consciousness is a quantum phenomenon, and have compared its behaviour to that of an electron at the subatomic level.

'The rule is, jam tomorrow and jam yesterday – but never jam to-day.'
'It MUST come sometimes to "jam to-day,"' Alice objected.
'No, it can't,' said the Queen.
'It's jam every OTHER day: to-day isn't any OTHER day, you know.'
'I don't understand you,' said Alice. 'It's dreadfully confusing!'
'That's the effect of living backwards,' the Queen said kindly: 'it always makes one a little giddy at first—'
'Living backwards!' Alice repeated in great astonishment. 'I never heard of such a thing!'
'—but there's one great advantage in it, that one's memory works both ways.'
'I'm sure MINE only works one way,' Alice remarked. 'I can't remember things before they happen.'
'It's a poor sort of memory that only works backwards,' the Queen remarked.

All matter at the subatomic level exists in wave form. That matter only appears solid when the brain decodes what it perceives and gives it form. Physicist Werner Heisenberg said, "What we observe is not nature itself, but nature exposed to our method of questioning."

Thoughts also exist in wave form. When they behave as a wave, they may leave the brain, existing outside the human mind, which would explain OBEs and NDEs. Quantum physics therefore suggests that consciousness is similar to the awareness an electron acquires when being observed – by a human – in the double slit experiment. So if an electron changes once it has been measured, perhaps a thought which has been "measured" or focused on may also cause the brain to behave differently. If, then, our perception of reality is governed by our brain, then the thoughts-become-things theory starts to look less improbable.

If the brain is in control of how we perceive reality, and if the entire universe is made up of atoms – with electrons inside them in a wave/particle dual state – then the mind can have some effect on our physical world. If we give our attention to certain thoughts while clearing out others, the networks we create will affect what 'happens' in our reality.

If this is true, it's a great way of no longer being the victim of circumstance.

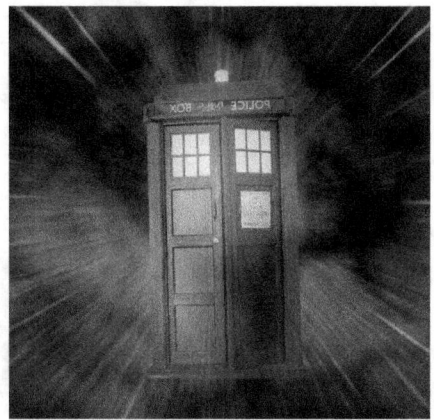

Visualising health, vitality and eternal youthfulness is not a fairy tale. Atoms are 99.9999% empty space and energy. Why then are we paying so much attention to the physical? Are we forgetting something?

Photo Credit: aussiegall via Compfight cc

Testosterone Levels

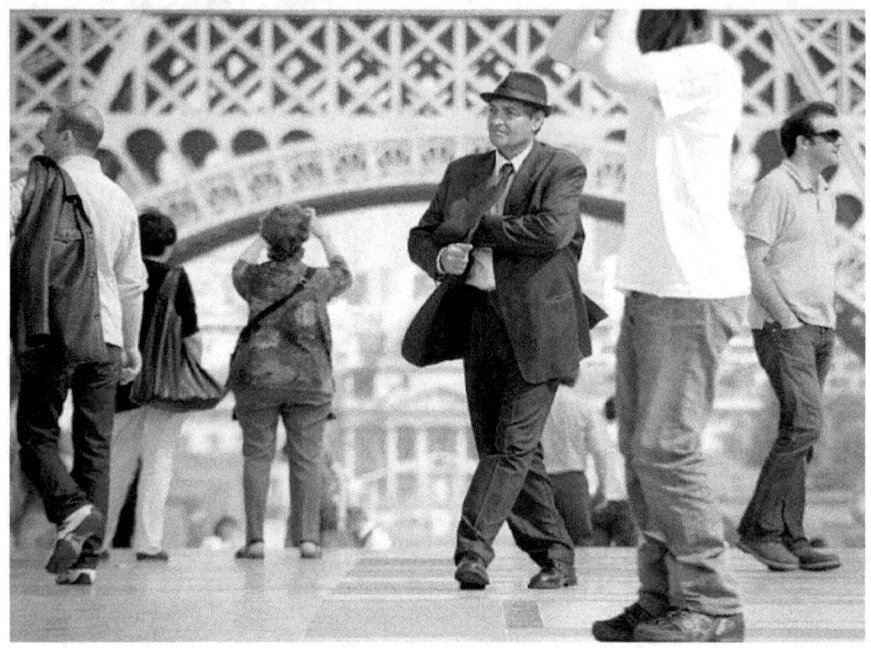

It has been assumed, for many years, that testosterone levels in men peak during the teen and early adult years, and then fall off by about 1% a year after age 30.

Or do they?

Testosterone is often associated with manhood, playing a major role in fertility and sexual prowess. It governs hair growth, red blood production, muscle and bone density and even emotional health. Scientists have some great news for mature men. Testosterone does not necessarily fall with age. It all comes down – once again – to health. A study done by the University of Adelaide on 1500 men between 35 and 80 found no significant difference in testosterone levels of healthy men. However,

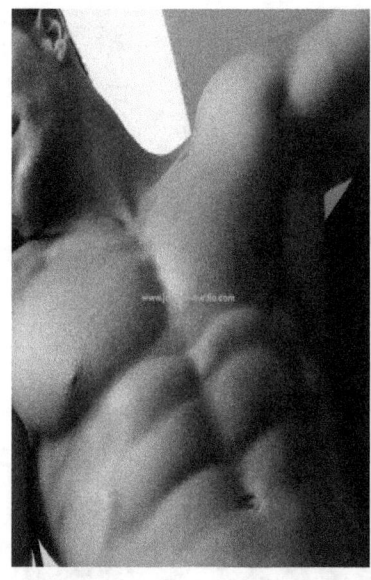

conditions such as obesity, depression and habits such as smoking did have a significant effect on the hormone. Evidence that testosterone is connected to well-being was also suggested by the fact men in a stable relationship had higher levels – this was thought to be not just because they got more sex, but because they were happier and healthier.

Another factor in the drop in testosterone levels was chemical exposure. Herbicides and statin drugs have been found to interfere with the testicles' ability to produce testosterone. This is one of the first studies that has followed the same group of men over time. The message for doctors is clear: a drop in testosterone in older men is not caused by ageing, but by diseases associated with ageing, which can be overcome and avoided.

"I've always suspected this," said one woman. "My husband is just as uncommunicative and bad-tempered at 80 as he was at 30."

Photo Credit: www.joaquin-murillo.com via Compfight cc
Photo Credit: Gregory Bastien via Compfight cc

The Vibe of Youth

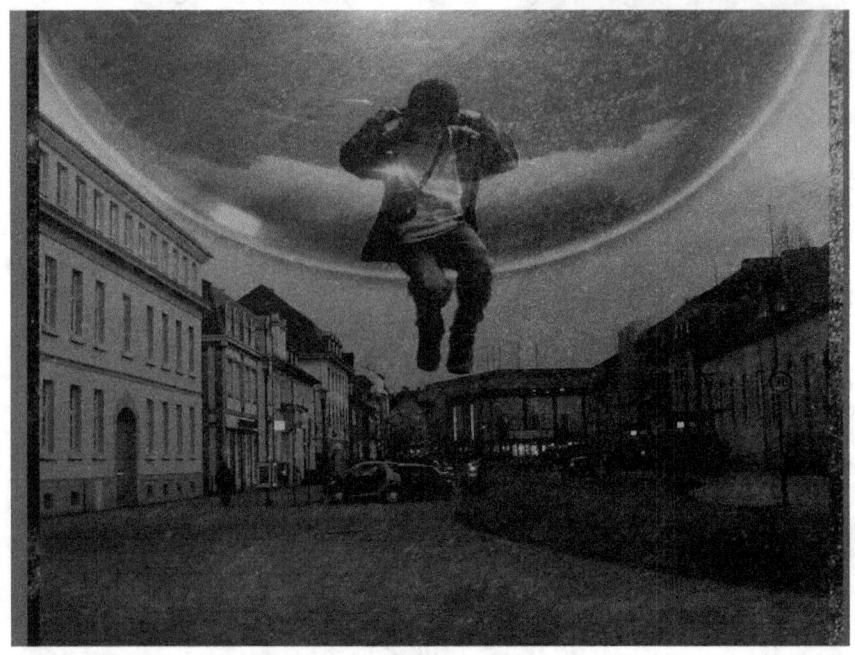

Although most people say inside they're the same now as they were at any age, consciousness does change, if only because of the expectations we have of what is still to come. It is now well established that people suffering from multiple personalities experience physical changes that accompany the mental switch. The most obvious and dramatic change is in voice quality, but there are other measurable differences such as visual acuity, ocular tension, corneal curvature, asthma, allergies, immune function and medication response (www.dissociative-identity-disorder.org).

Someone who is at the beginning of their life may not imagine they will one day be fearing decline, and someone who is 'over the hill' of retirement age, or getting there, has perhaps forgotten what it is

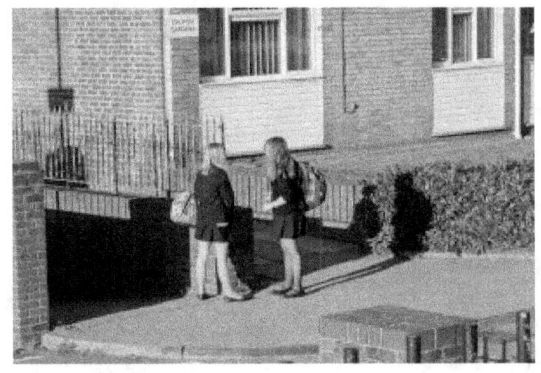 to feel they have their whole life ahead of them. It is this feeling of potential that keeps us young, and as we have all been young, it can be brought again to the surface with a simple mindfulness technique.

Our thoughts and emotions are crucial to epigenetic changes in our bodies, and so learning to recapture the vibration of youth can make a huge difference to our health and well-being, as well as our appearance and lifespan. This simple meditation can be adapted by anyone to bring back not only the pictures, but the sensations, emotions and essential vibe of youth.

Let us with closed eyes cast our mind back to our schooldays.

Let us feel the sensation of being back in that building, sense the light from another time streaming back through the windows.

We picture ourselves in a classroom, with a memorable teacher.

Who is sitting around us? Recall those personalities.

What are we wearing? Feel the sensation of the material between our fingers, the pen in our pencil case, the smells of chalk dust, rubber and fresh photocopy ink, the school bag (what is inside?) Do we recall the colour of the school books? The form of our handwriting?

What smells are there? Mown grass? Canteen smells? The smell of chalk dust, an eraser, the wood of the desk?

Look at the desk – what marks are there? Recall the colour and shape of the chair. What sounds are there? Cries from another classroom? The bell signalling a change of class? The sound of a sports game in the field? The voice of a teacher? What subject are we learning? Are we straining to understand what may now seem easy? Is it boring, fascinating, or easy? What school trips, holidays or leisure activities are we looking forward to? Recapture those feelings of confidence or frustration.

Visualise a small area in the building. A corner by the radiator? The pile of exercise books on the teacher's desk? A window with a view in the stairwell? Try and recall as many details as possible.

What are we working towards? A test? A national exam? What are our primary emotions? A crush on a teacher or another student? Are we smarting from a hurtful comment? What complexes do we have, and what fears? How do we feel about going home to our families when the day is over? What is the weather like as we walk back home? Is it a winter's day, the light already fading? Or is the heat of the day still strong? Feel what it is to have a young body, and above all a young face. Recall the onset of menstruation for women, the rising sexual power of the adolescent boy. Do we feel attractive or ungainly? What are our hopes? How did we feel about future employment or college, how did we imagine it before we found out what it really was like? Sense the anticipation and uncertainty of that time.

Now sink deeper and deeper into the vibration of youth until we feel we really are our younger selves. We stay with that vibration for as long as feels natural before rising up to the present time, with the sensation still with us.

Is Happiness Fleeting?

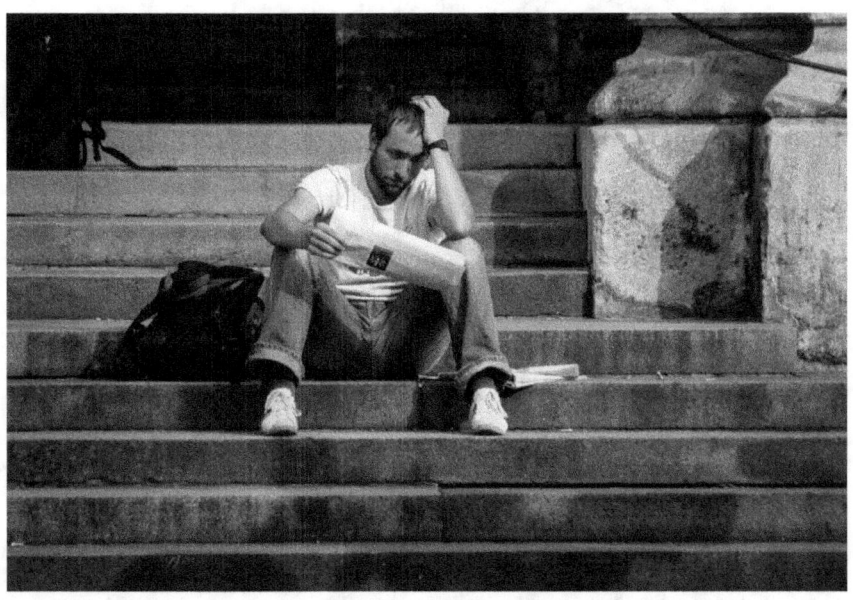

It is said that happiness lasts about fifteen minutes. Sooner or later either some news will arrive to spoil it or a niggling thought will surface to change it. Even when we are happy, we worry about what might take our happiness away. Happiness is not stationary. It is always moving. No matter what we get or achieve, happiness from external events will be short-lived. Successful people who have achieved their goal report immediately focusing on the next one. It is human nature to always be looking for the next big thing. There is nothing wrong with that. Life would be dull if we had nothing to look forward to, so the question is, how can we change our set point and get happiness to last?

In a classic study conducted by the Southern Methodist University, three groups were given a writing task. One was asked to spend a few minutes over four days describing their ideal future, another

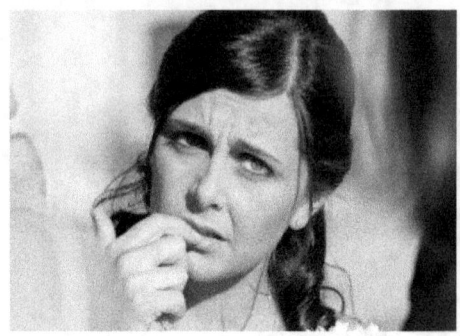 had to describe their plans for the day and the third was asked to relate a traumatic event. The results revealed that the happiest group, even three months later, were those who described intense happiness in the future; they reported longer periods of contentedness during the day. Although talking about trauma felt cathartic at the time, it did not have any long-lasting effect on happiness itself. The key with discussing trauma seems to be to release the feelings and replace them with positive thoughts that the trauma is dealt with, that wisdom has been gained through the experience. Simply replaying it in our minds will reproduce the feelings of despair the original event provoked.

Feeling unhappy is more often than not a result of thinking about past unhappiness or imagining a bleak future. When asked what makes them unhappy a group of people replied :

- Remembering loved ones they had lost through death or separation
- Recalling feelings of hope that were dashed
- Remembering a moment of intense shame or defeat
- Feeling unloved, unwanted, rejected
- Worrying about loneliness
- Dissatisfaction with work and relationships

Dwelling on these things causes a drop in serotonin, which affects mood, creating a vicious circle of sadness. Action is needed to reverse mood, and force of will to play an upbeat piece of music for example, when we feel a sad melody would better match our state of mind. Medical conditions that cause depression such as thyroid imbalances may be originally caused by stress, and stress is a result of our perception of our circumstances.
Counting our blessings may seem a twee response to an apparently desperate status quo. Humans have a tendency to focus on the

negative however, in a misguided attempt to avoid denial. But we can be aware of an issue without allowing it to alter our perception of life. Whatever problems we face, there are always others who have it worse; there is always something to feel thankful for.

Homes for the elderly are full of people still fretting after all these years. Let us not die worrying about the future.

Photo Credit: spaceodissey via Compfight cc
Photo Credit: mohammadali via Compfight cc

Come again?

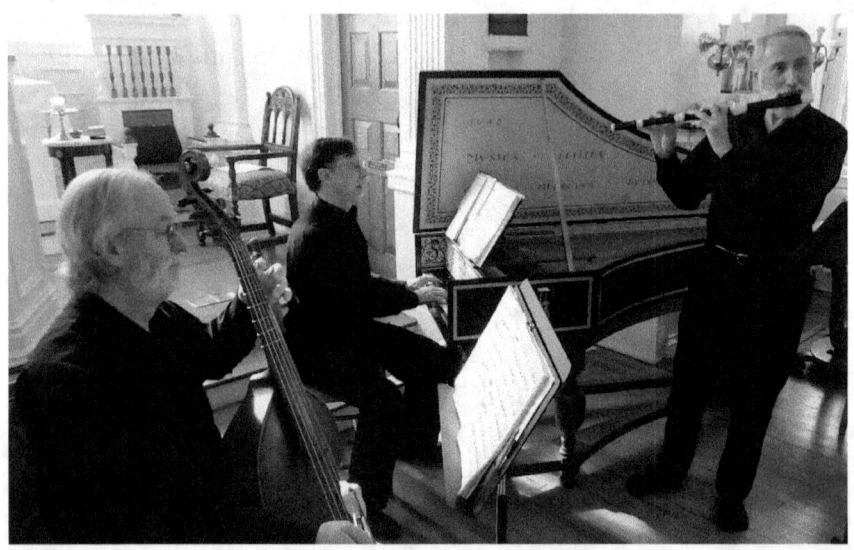

Hearing begins to deteriorate in our twenties. There are internet hearing tests available which give our hearing age. Over 30% of people above age 60 and over 50% of people above age 85 have hearing loss. Hearing loss is a serious issue, not simply because it makes life difficult but because of the consequences for our brain. Mature adults with impaired hearing may have a faster rate of brain shrinkage, since the ear is no longer sending clear messages to the brain. Without that input, sound-processing brain regions may change in structure and lead to a decline in memory and thinking skills.

Hearing loss is due to damage to the tiny hairs in the ear responsible for transmitting sound to the brain and to the nerves which govern hearing. Other causes include diabetes, exposure to loud noises, medication, smoking and genetics.

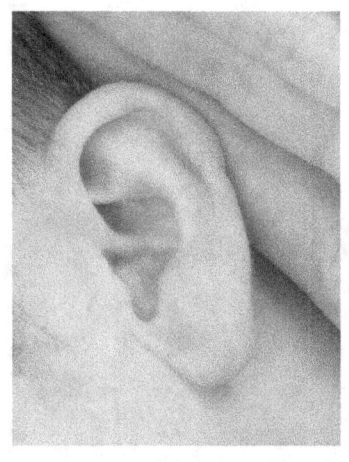

If we find ourselves frequently asking people to repeat themselves, have difficulty in understanding high voices and the difference between 's' and 'th', and if we experience problems in focusing on a conversation in a crowded area, hearing loss may have begun. However, all is not lost. There are ways to prevent further deterioration and even reverse it. We can train our ears to distinguish sound more easily by listening to classical music since it uses a variety of noise levels and frequencies. Those with hearing loss show vitamin deficiencies, but studies have shown hearing can be improved by ensuring we have a sufficient amount of B12, vitamins C, D and E, folic acid and zinc. Magnesium (contained in almonds, cashews, peanuts, spinach, yoghurt....) has been repeatedly demonstrated to reverse noise-induced hearing loss.

The brain is constantly creating neurons. Experiments done on adult mice kept in the dark show their hearing improves due to the strengthening of connections between neurons, a development normally only occurring in childhood. Visual impairment in humans improves cognition of pitch and frequency, which proves that intervention can alter hearing efficiency.

Calorie restriction has also been demonstrated to reduce the incidence of age-related hearing loss. Blood sugar control, proper nutrition and avoiding exposure to loud sounds can all help in preventing a silent old age. Come again?

Photo Credit: Photos by Mavis via Compfight cc

Cellular Memory

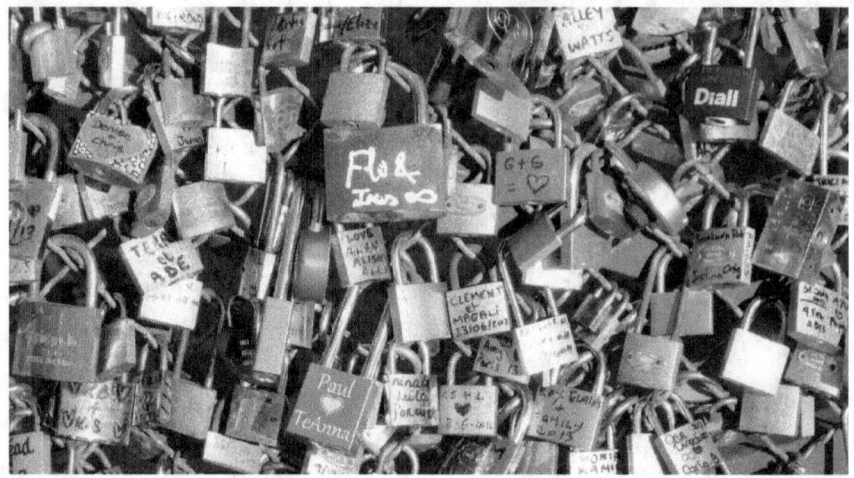

In many native cultures, eating the heart of your enemy was said to allow you to absorb his courage and strength. Bizarrely this belief may have some basis in fact. The controversy surrounding cellular memory is fading away. Until quite recently claims that memories can be stored in places other than the brain were discounted as evidence of scientific illiteracy, a lack of critical thinking skills and downright gullibility. But the idea has progressed from the category of pseudoscience to that of a valid theory, and evidence continues to emerge that cellular memory is a reality.

On a daily basis, cellular memory may be the cause of sudden, inexplicable pains – or "phantom pains" – in parts of the body that seem otherwise healthy. We may be tempted to put them down to ageing, but it is worth examining the thoughts and circumstances that preceded the expression of the pain to determine whether they were related to a physically or emotionally traumatic event.

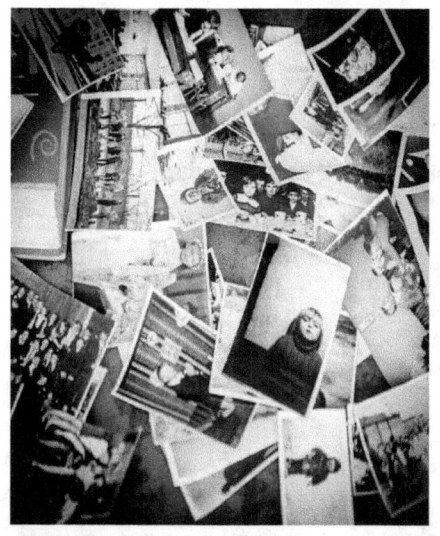

Undigested trauma as a result of intentional repression, a sense of helplessness due to past abuse or feelings of embarrassment, shame and rage that linger long after the event may all cause disease. The theory is that neuropeptides, which send messages through the body, lock onto cells through the cell receptor sites. The types of neuropeptides flowing through the body depend on our different emotional states throughout the day. Viruses also enter the cell through these receptor sites, and if the receptor for the natural peptide (expressing for example fear, or guilt) is present in enough numbers, viruses which match will have an easier time getting into the cell. The peptides for negative emotions can also block the entry into the cell for the messengers that keep the body functioning properly. This is why stress reduction is as important if not more important than healthy eating, for if the nutrients cannot enter the cell in the first place, our body will eventually fall ill.

However long ago the traumatic event was, the emotion will be on hold as long as it is not resolved. And if we accept the theory of the holographic universe, it may be that the entire personality is contained in each group of cells and is perpetuated even when these cells are renewed.

Major organs such as the lungs, heart and kidneys have a large number of neural networks – self-contained 'brains' that may store a host of information. The reason why the idea that cells have memories is gaining support among scientists and medical practitioners is that there is an increasing body of evidence from the recipients of donor organs. Following the transplant, many patients have reported changes in food preferences, music, literature tastes and in their personalities.

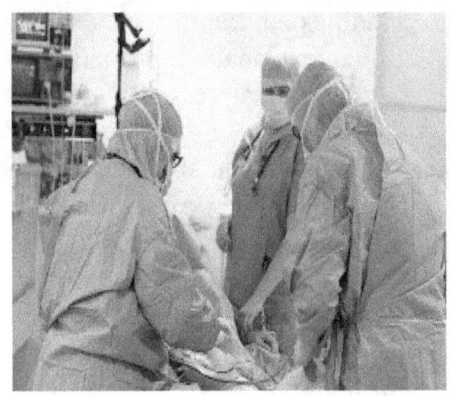

Claire Sylvia, a 47 yr-old American woman, was one of the first to report this odd phenomenon in 1988. After receiving a heart and lung transplant she claimed to crave beer and chicken nuggets, things she did not enjoy before. She later discovered her donor was an 18 yr-old boy killed in a motorcycle accident. His family confirmed his love for beer and that chicken nuggets were his favourite food.

Bill Wohl received a heart transplant in 2000 after suffering from cardiac disease. A tough 'type A' executive, he reacted emotionally to a song on the radio by Sade weeks after the surgery. The crying and rocking was so extreme he contacted the family of his donor, a 36 yr-old Hollywood stuntman, and discovered Sade was one of his favourite singers. Wohl had never heard of Sade before.

A woman who was terrified of heights until she was given the lungs of a mountain climber also experienced a life-changing experience.

Dottie O'Connor from Massachusetts is now a climber too. Sonny Graham from South Carolina, who received the lungs of a man who committed suicide and subsequently married his widow, later also committed suicide, leaving the wife to grieve all over again. Both Terry Cottle and Sonny Graham shot themselves at an interval of twelve years. Friends of Mr Graham said he had shown no signs of being depressed.

Cheryl Johnson from Lancashire used to enjoy celebrity biographies and best sellers such as *The Da Vinci Code*. But following a kidney transplant she prefers classics such as Jane Austen's *Persuasion* and Dostoevsky's *Crime and Punishment*.

Paul Oldam, a lawyer from Milwaukee, received the heart of a 14-year-old boy and inherited his craving for Snickers.

The body's cellular memory can be accessed through deep meditation or with a kinesiologist. A dialogue is established involving mind and body. The link between the conscious and the unconscious mind and gentle manipulation known as muscle testing can be used to identify trapped cellular memories and/or physical disease. By systematically questioning areas of the body the therapist can home in on the problem and direct healing to that area.

Sceptics speculate that the patient unconsciously hears doctors and nurses talking about the donor while under anesthesia and somehow is suggestible. Any subsequent personality change could therefore be due to unconscious feelings of sympathy and gratitude or guilt. But the cellular memory phenomenon is too becoming too widespread for us to ignore. Let's not stew in our own juice. Accessing our body's cellular memory may release trapped trauma and eliminate disease waiting to happen.

Is it unnatural to wish to stay ageless?

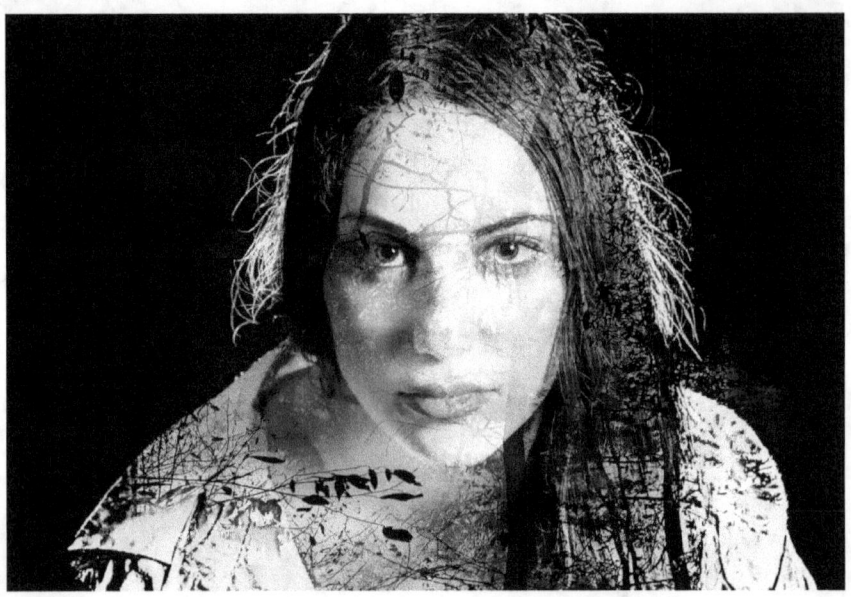

One of the most compelling arguments about the fight to conquer ageing is that it is unnatural. Those who believe this feel that trying to beat nature at its game is not only perverse, but could lead to boredom when life outlives its value, that it brings about social inequity when poor people die younger while the rich and educated find ways of prolonging life and that it exacerbates prejudice against the old by deifying the young and healthy. In Greek mythology, Tithonus was a beautiful youth and lover of Eos the goddess of the Dawn. Eos asked Zeus to grant him immortality but forgot to request eternal youth, so that Tithonus was condemned to age forever. Eventually Eos hid him in a basket in despair.

Endless frailty is not what we are about. Staying ageless means just that – extending a healthy life. Most people would agree that it is a noble goal to seek to conquer the suffering caused by diseases such

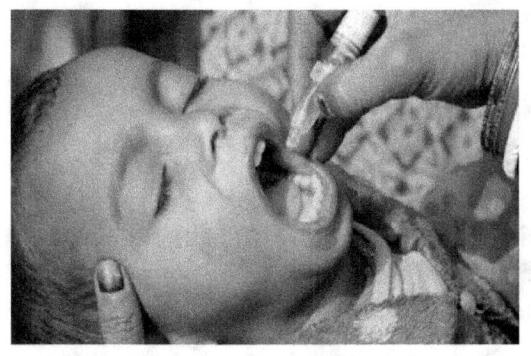 as cancer, Alzheimer's, arthritis, heart disease, stroke and the decline of hearing and vision. Curing these symptoms of ageing is never seen as reprehensible, and yet curing ageing itself is. But there are organisms in nature that do not age (tortoises, lobsters, hydra, rockfish). Moreover calorie restriction, a natural phenomenon during periods of famine, has been shown to prolong life in many organisms. Lifespan in humans has increased dramatically anyway, and the number of centenarians is climbing steadily without a specific "cure" having ever been announced. In any case no one would be forced to extend their life : if we are in favour of personal choice we must therefore also accept those among us who wish to maximise their lifespan.

Is it arrogant to wish to live longer? Some may claim it is playing God, but if that is true all research into heart disease, cancer and stroke should end now. Would it perpetuate and aggravate social injustice if life extension were to be available to a chosen, wealthy few? There are two arguments against this. Firstly, all medical advances are always initially available to a select few; this is true of vaccines, antibiotics and new medicines. Eventually their use becomes widespread. We do not halt chemotherapy because it is not available to everyone. Pioneers proceed regardless of whether there is world peace or an end to poverty, since progress eventually has spin-offs for all. The internet and mobile phones were invented in the West but now these are widely available in even the poorest nations. In fact overcoming the infirmity of ageing would have economic benefits for all governments who would no longer spend billions of dollars on health care for the elderly. Secondly, it is our belief that medical progress is not the whole story, probably not even the main part of it, and that there is a major spiritual, attitudinal component of seeking agelessness, since it may well involve practising moderation, balancing leisure and work, relaxation and exertion, and directing our emotions and thoughts – something which is available to everyone.

If we were to live completely natural lives, we would not have vaccination, or antibiotics, or any medicine at all. If we were living the natural life, there would be no farming, TV, computers or transport other than by horse. Likewise there would be no contraception, and many women would die in childbirth. Those who did not would give birth without pain relief, and suffer mentally with fear of death at each new pregnancy. Unplanned children would suffer emotionally. There would be no sanitation and cholera would kill 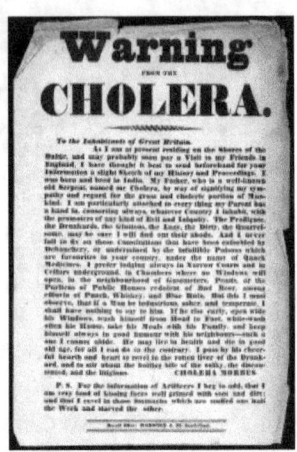 thousands every year. Natural selection would reign supreme; there would be no care for the disabled, and those of us who have suffered broken limbs would be permanently maimed. In the 1918 flu epidemic, the virus was most lethal for those in the prime of life. 99% of deaths were in people under 65. The virus is thought to have caused an overreaction of the immune systems of healthy young adults. In the first 25 weeks Spanish flu killed 25 million people worldwide – a purely natural phenomenon.

Is it ethically reprehensible to wish to end ageing? We would argue it is reprehensible not to end suffering, and if we do not take action, we are all condemned to suffer some symptom of old age. Some authors have argued it is morally wrong to wish to extend life, but as we have been doing precisely that for hundreds of years, according to this argument we are all living immoral lives already.

A True Present

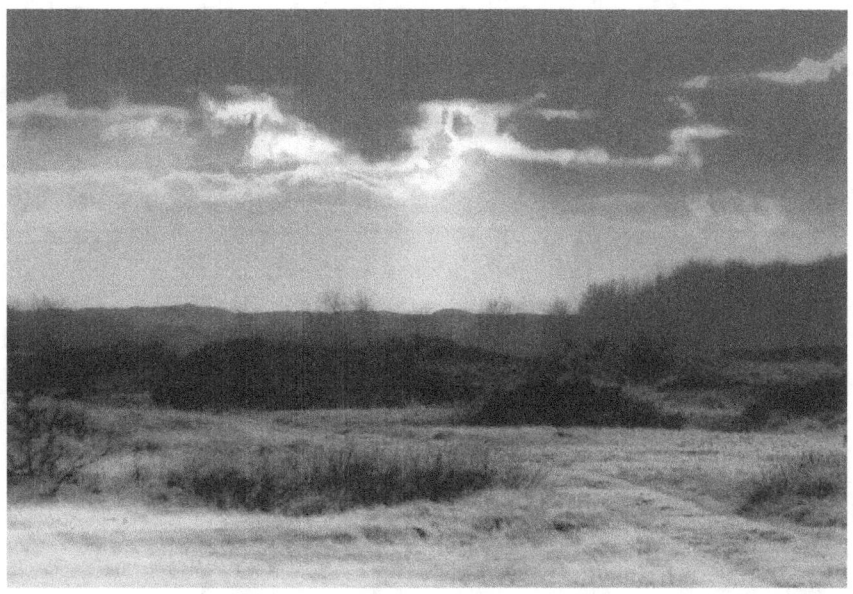

Many people say time speeds up as we age. The long summer holidays of childhood seemed to be endless, but as our minds filled with more and more concerns, life began to rush by. As we age we find ourselves spending less and less time in the present. Wouldn't it be wonderful if we could spend our lives, from now on, without worrying, but instead truly experiencing every moment life lays before us?

Experiencing a true present is something most of us find difficult. Even when on holiday we often find miles of countryside have slipped by unseen while we focus on our inner chatter, consisting of plans and past regrets and reliving scenes of our lives, or analysing people's motives and intentions. The overactive mind is often seen as a scourge of Western culture, but the Oriental mind is just as susceptible to overload. A Tai Chi master from a Beijing

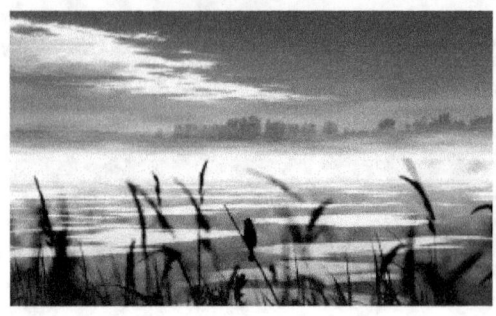 martial arts school was asked if she drifted off during her movements to think about having forgotten to pop into the bank. She replied that although she manages to be totally into her routine thanks to her training, she has noticed that since the advent of the car, people in China are also beginning to fall victim to a racing mind and an addiction to getting ahead. "It was better when we had bicycles," she said. "People were more mindful. They would step back and let others pass. They were more aware of the day as it passed."

An overactive mind can hinder us from getting enough sleep and in its worst forms is a symptom of hypermania. Racing thoughts can prevent us from focusing on one topic or activity; they tire us out, increase anxiety, cause stress and increase the speed at which we live – and age. Slow breathing, writing out thoughts, exercise or mindfulness meditation can all help to slow us down and bring focus. When the moment we are in is a painful one, then we can direct the mind and the body towards more peaceful thoughts by breathing through the pain and remembering that everything must pass. The worst scenario is that we will never feel good again; now how likely is that?

It is part of the human condition to have an active mind, but it is also part of our heritage to be able to still that mind and focus on the now. Once broken, the habit of constantly worrying and projecting will soon begin to fade and it is never too late, whatever our culture and heritage. We must remember that in the spiritual life we are always at the beginning, whoever we are.

Shall we have our bath now?

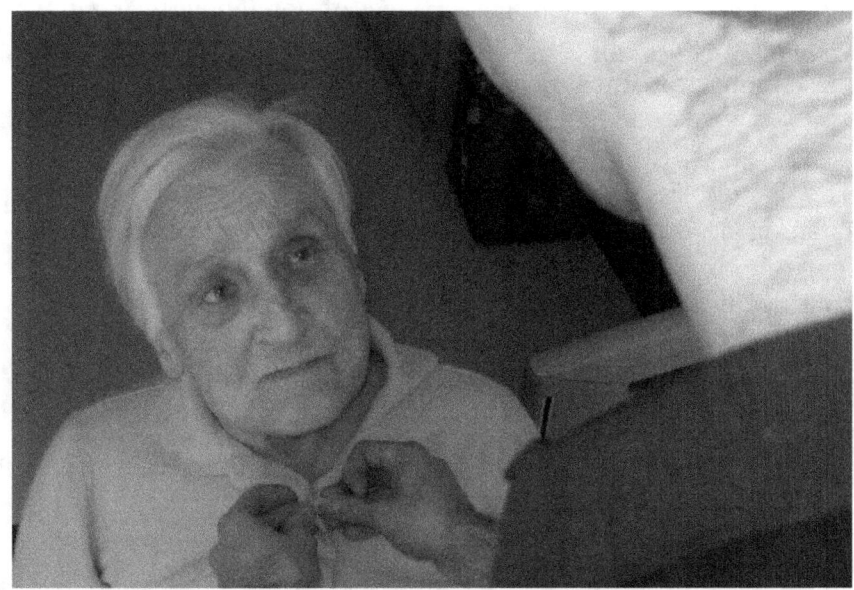

We live in an ageist society. Ageism arises from a set of beliefs predicated on the assumption of biological and cognitive decline in older people. It is manifest in the media, which often places the elderly alongside other groups which suffer from deprivation and prejudice such as the disabled and ethnic minorities, and in corporate and social attitudes that perpetuate the idea that older people must be treated differently, depicting them in cartoons and advertisements as being on a par with children, or categorising them as either dirty old men or wicked witches. Some social theories exacerbate these attitudes, such as Disengagement Theory (Cummin/Henry), which states that death is least disruptive to social harmony if older people have first disengaged from society and relationships before they die. The archetype of the helpless, infantile old man or woman sometimes produces instances of elder abuse, or 'granny battering', which can vary from violence and financial exploitation to more subtle forms such as infantilisation in the way seniors are addressed and treated. Continuing to work after retirement sometimes comes up against disapproval fueled by the argument it is time for them to move over and free up jobs for the young, but it is often the very fact of continuing to work and making a contribution to society that protects older people from these forms of maltreatment.

The more blatant forms of elder abuse are easy to spot, but infantilising adults through intonation and puerile group activities is more difficult to address, since it can have the veneer of consideration and care. Infantilising intonation is something community elders are particularly resentful of since it smacks of disrespect, and there is no evidence it produces a sense of care and concern.

Infantilisation of older people may include:

- Activities more appropriate to primary school, such as colouring, being asked to name favourite foods or animals, recalling early childhood memories and circulating bright pictures of feast days such as Valentine's Day or Christmas.
- Responding to problems as though talking to a child, ("I just changed you and you wet your diaper again!" instead of, "I'll change your briefs if that's all right." Or "Now now, let's not be lazy, next time make sure you ring the bell," and other demeaning put-downs.)
- Using terms such as "poppet" and "dear" and the moronic interrogative when explaining medical procedures, i.e. upward intonation at the end of a sentence turning a statement into a question, implying the hearer may be incapable of understanding.
- Authoritarian body language – scowls, pointing, and other gestures that express irritation.

- Non-speech sounds intended to berate – tuts, whistles and hums.
- Selecting 'appropriate' TV entertainment, or ending discussions on adult subjects such as sex in a school mistressy manner.
- Talking about a person in their presence as if they were absent.
- Parenting attitudes such as withdrawal of privileges for bad behaviour or threats, "If you don't take your medication you can't go to bingo."
- Using the first person plural as in, "Shall we have our bath now?"

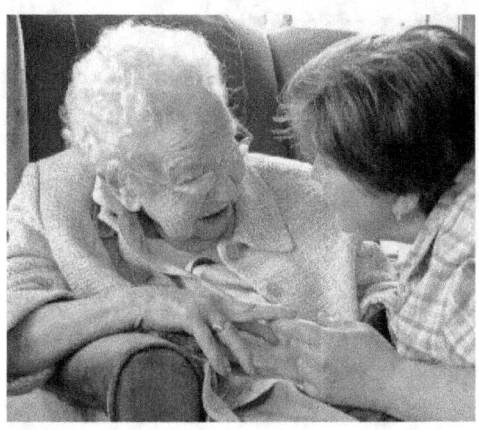

These subtle forms of abuse encourage disengagement and dependency. Nursing staff, carers and family members report stress, burn-out and overwork as the reasons for these slips. But we will all one day reach our golden years and must think of how we would wish to be treated. Infantilising older people contributes to a sense of hopelessness and can hasten cognitive and physical decline. Older adults, with or without dementia, deserve respect, to be addressed as 'Mr Smith', as we would any younger person. Otherwise, what goes around comes around.

Photo Credit: McBeth via Compfight cc

The Tree of Life

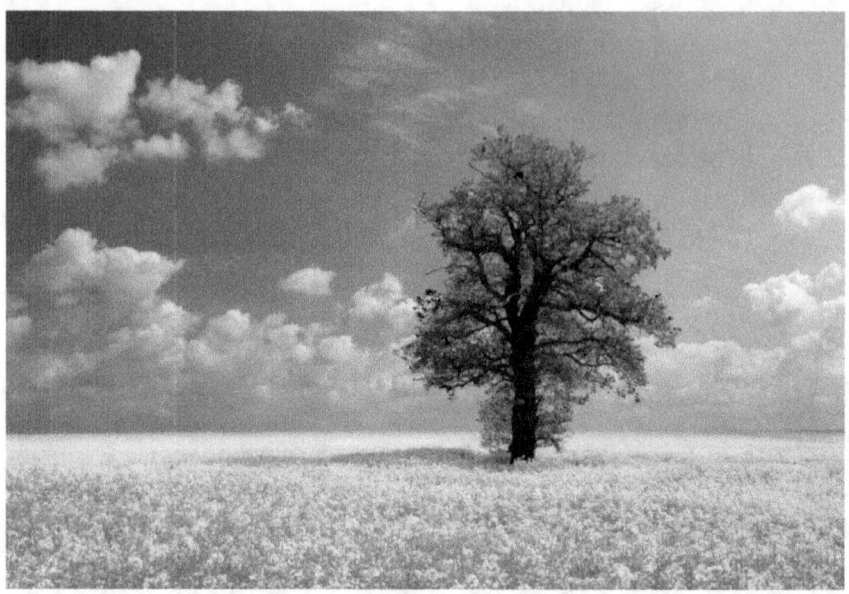

Sometimes called the cosmic or world tree, the tree of life did not originate with the authors of Genesis. The notion of a sacred tree appears in many traditions. Isis and Osiris were said to have emerged from an acacia tree, which the Egyptians considered to be the tree of life. The Mayan tree of life is a cross from which branches emerge, the centre of which symbolises the point of absolute beginning, the source of all creation. The oldest name of Babylon (Tintirki) meant the place of the tree of life. This was a tree with magical fruit which could be picked only by the gods. Sumerian art depicts it guarded by a pair of intertwined snakes. In the Book of Revelation the tree of life is described as having curative properties ("And the leaves of the tree are for the healing of the nations" – Revelation 22:2). Consider also the Buddha who received enlightenment under the Bodhi tree.

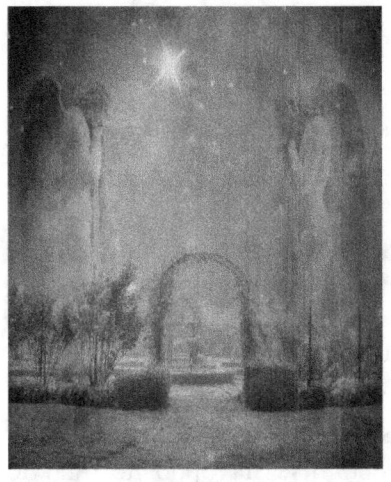

It is clear that the symbol of immortality and freedom from all disease is an archetype deeply embedded in the human consciousness. A tree has deep connections with the earth, yet its branches reach up to heaven. It symbolises a link between the material and the metaphysical world.

However as we all know, in the Garden of Eden alongside the tree of life was another tree: the tree of the knowledge of good and evil. Adam and Eve fell out of favour with God by eating its fruit, and were cast out of the garden, condemned to toil all their lives and to experience illness, ageing and death. In one of the scriptural writings outside the Canon (*Vita Adae et Evae*), as Adam lies ill and dying his son Seth is described asking him what pain is, and Adam explains it is a result of the knowledge of good and evil. He expresses feelings of guilt, and begs his son to go back into Eden to get oil from the tree of life to relieve his suffering, but to no avail. To prevent access to this tree in the future Genesis says that cherubim with flaming swords flashing back and forth were placed at the garden's entrance to guard the way.

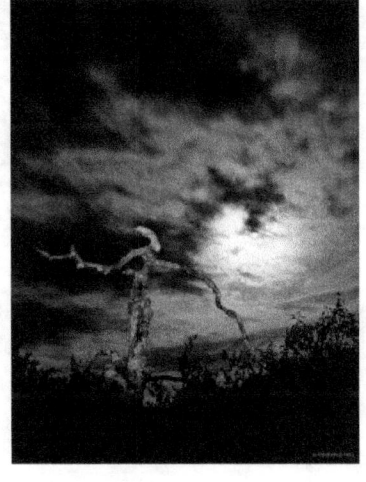

The theological explanation for why a loving God would allow death is that because of sin, life is filled with pain, illness and hard work, and by limiting our lifespan God spares us the misery of an endless existence full of suffering and heartache. The wages of sin, as St Paul says, is death, but God allows us to reach out to him and offers eternal life after death through Christ.

Why does the Bible call the second of these trees the tree of the knowledge of good and evil instead of just calling it the tree of death? It is as though knowledge of good and evil is equated with the opposite of life. This rather confusing message can be interpreted in two ways. The standard theological interpretation is that knowing good and evil meant experiencing it, and that the sin of man condemned him to suffer evil and pain, so that he might better appreciate what is good and true. It is certainly the case that for many metaphysical philosophies, one of the explanations for suffering is that it enables us to recognise its opposite, and to expand our consciousness in order to acquire greater wisdom. But if we take this analogy further, we can apply the word 'knowledge' to all of the information that our minds soak up from the time we are born on earth. Much of this information serves as a source of social cues, beliefs and learned thought patterns, causing us to

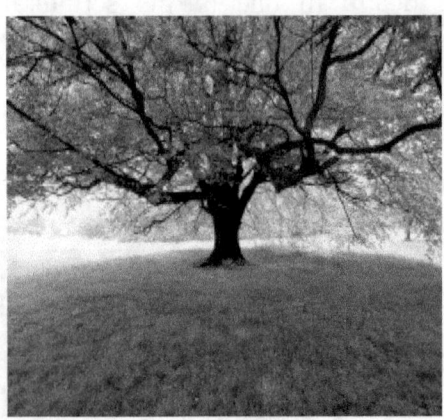

adopt unconscious attitudes towards health and human lifespan that set our inner clock to begin to age at a given time, and leading us to associate pain and fatigue with advancing years, as well as constantly calculating how long we have left. Cognition is not a representation of the world, but an interpretation of it.

In the Kabbalah, 'Ain Soph' is beyond good and evil, embracing the totality of everything. It may be translated as 'there is no end' or 'infinite' and represents the divine origin of all created existence. It emanates 10 realms of existence, the lowest of which is the realm of our universe. Ain Soph has parallels in science : in the case of string theory, consistency requires space-time to have 10 dimensions.

Daring to turn our back on the 'knowledge of good and evil' and associating ourselves with the tree of life, clearing our minds of negative chatter and filling our lives with the positive, the uplifting, with affirming statements rather than thinking about what we don't want, don't have and need to resist, is a step few would call rational, but there are already many who are edging their way back into the garden through conscious living, as the flaming swords are lowered and Eden comes again into sight.

<u>Things We Regret At The End</u>

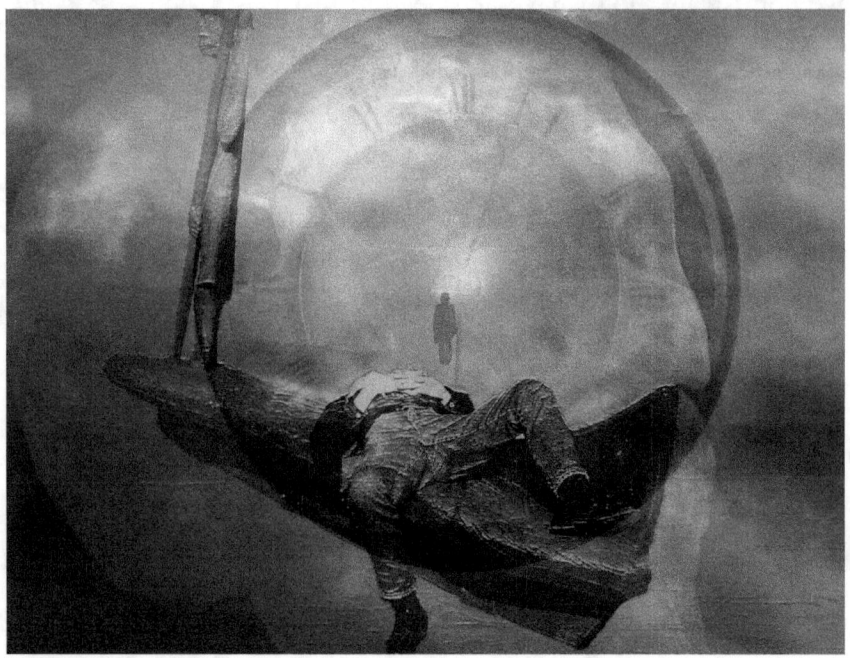

Nurses in palliative care report that there is a pattern to the things people nearing the end of their lives regret. They won't all apply to us, but among this list is surely at least one lesson for those of us with some time left – and that means everyone who is not going to die within the next few minutes.

I wish :

- I'd had more time – it is important to experience the present fully, to savour the sights and smells and emotions and the laughter and words of our peers.
- I hadn't worried so much – in retrospect why did we make such a fuss a few years ago? The same will apply to today's worries in the future.
- I'd appreciated what I had. We can start doing this today.
- I'd examined and eliminated more of my faults and learnt more wisdom. A spiritual approach to life, examining how we could have dealt with situations differently does not mean we have to be religious.
- I'd spent more time with my family and friends rather than at work and recovering from fatigue.
- I hadn't taken myself so seriously – laughing at ourselves is a virtue.
- I'd done more for others – helping others and sharing what life has given us, whether this be possessions or abilities, gives life meaning.
- I could have felt happier – when we are at the end of our lives we realise happiness is a state of mind. Happiness is a choice.
- I'd cared less what other people think. When we realise how little people think about us we are free to live our lives as we wish. How much do we think about other people's choices? Would we be surprised if they were affected by our opinion? Being a people pleaser does not lead to personal fulfilment.
- I'd taken more risks. Think of all the long dead people who lived their lives being very, very careful. Were they right? What if they had done something unusual instead? Which sort of person do we like to read about today?
- I'd taken better care of myself. What would we be like today if we had started really looking after our health 30 years ago? Ignoring our health, particularly among men, is one of the top regrets.
- I'd trusted my gut instead of listening to everyone else and followed my passion in life. Wishing we'd accomplished more is the most common regret of all. Unfulfilled dreams leave a bitter taste on the deathbed.

- I'd worked less – financial success isn't the key to a happy life. By simplifying life it is possible to live more and work less. How might I not need so much money? And if we hate our job, this is even more true.
- I'd told him/her what I truly felt – for good or for bad, bringing closure and eliminating negative cellular memory, since bitterness and resentment can lead to disease. Even though the person's reaction may be nuclear, it raises the relationship to a new, healthier level or allows the relationship to fade away.
- I hadn't let good friendships slip and hadn't hung on to friendships that had run their course out of a sense of duty or courtesy. The physical details of life slip away when we are faced with our mortality and we remember what people gave or took away from us.
- I hadn't got married early; as the years pass spouses often have different ideas of how their relationship should evolve. Everyone who gets out of a bad relationship regrets not getting out earlier.
- I'd used sunscreen. 90% of wrinkles are caused by the sun.
- I'd realised how good-looking I was. Let's take a look at a photo of ourselves 20 years ago. Now what were we worried about?
- I hadn't held onto grudges. Waste of time. Let go and move on.
- I'd stood up for myself. Saying 'back off', or if we can't because it's the boss, 'that's a very harsh comment' eliminates endless replaying of injustices. This ability often comes with experience.
- I hadn't neglected my teeth. Floss, floss, floss.

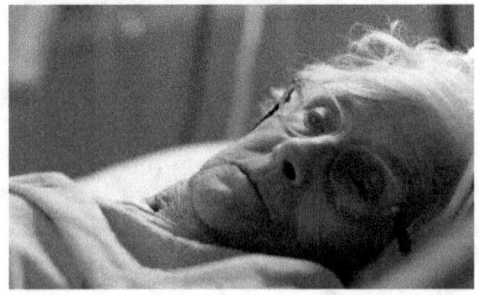

It's never too late to change. While we are still standing, let's make a move. Imagine we're on our death bed now – what life would we like to look back on?

And finally…in a TV interview he gave in his old age, poet John Betjeman was asked the conventional question: "Do you have any regrets?" Replied the poet: "Yes. I wish I'd had more sex."

The Power of Perception

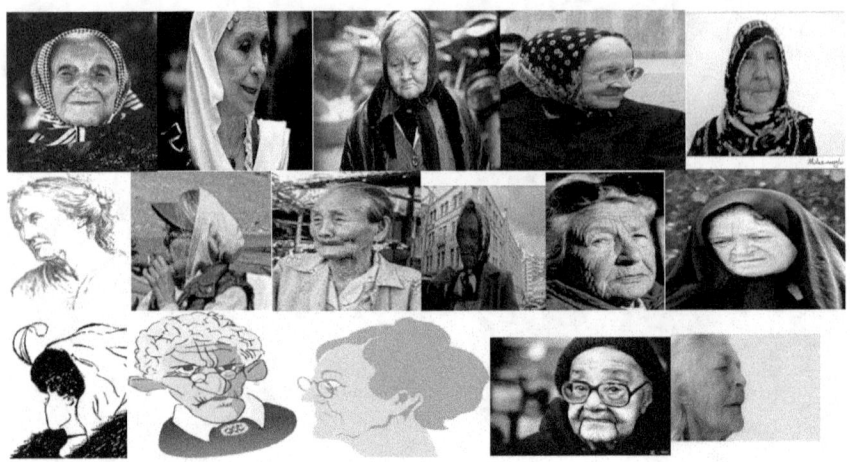

The atmosphere was souring by the minute. One woman's perception was that the school was doing its best, that there were far worse situations in other schools, in other areas of the country, and that more discipline would lead to abuse. The other woman

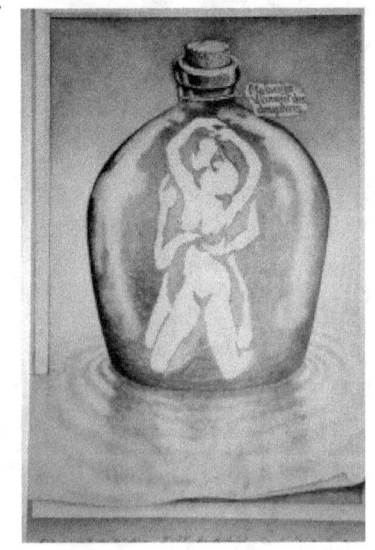

snorted with disdain at the degree of ignorance in this perception. Letting children run wild in a school was the reason why society was going to the dogs. The implication in the argument was that one knew better how to raise children than the other. The atmosphere remained strained for the rest of the day.

What happens when we hear or see something unfamiliar? First we seek all the information we can detect, and want to learn more. Second we compare what we see with what we have seen and known in the past. Third we seek to categorise, accepting and rejecting different pieces of information through a process of increasingly intense selective filtering, until we hit upon a conclusion. Thus we categorise and interpret sensory information in a way that favours one interpretation over another. In the image of a vase young children see dolphins. Likewise, individuals reach different conclusions about media events according to their preconceived ideas. In this way an identical event may lead different political parties to adopt diametrically opposing views on action.

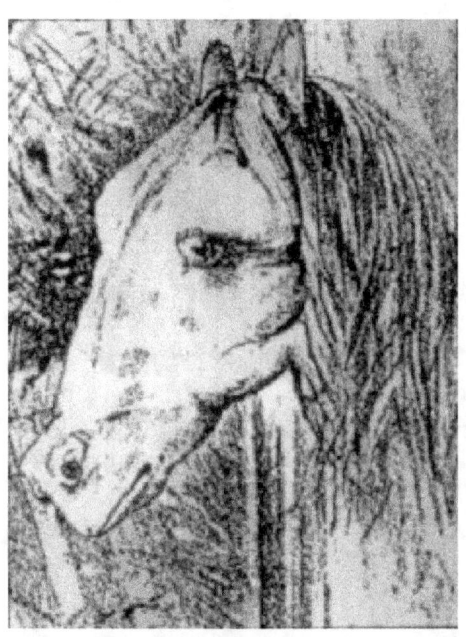

In one experiment, students told they were consuming alcohol became gradually more drunk in their behaviour, even though no alcohol was present. In another, subjects were given an article to read about flu and then shown pictures of people. They then identified possible carriers of the virus – who turned out to be obese people, foreigners and the elderly. Thus this image of a horse is not a horse at all when viewed sideways. The process of selective perception may also vary in the individual according to his or her prior emotional state. In related research, participants who had agreed to walk on their campus carrying a large, embarrassing sign underestimated the distance to be crossed. This was a result of trying to cope with the contradiction of doing something unpleasant of their own free will.

In fact the way the brain interprets stimuli cannot be trusted. If we plunge a cold hand into a bowl of lukewarm water it will feel warmer than if our hands were at room temperature.

Another example of how perceptions can vary can be found in language. We may listen to a foreign language and hear only the music and the sounds as a long, uninterrupted melody, but when we learn the language there is an Aha! moment as the sounds separate first into words and then into meaning. In the header image on the previous page, among the old women is a girl no more than twenty. When you spot her you will think again about helping her up the steps.

Each of us tends to believe our view of the world is the correct one, but this is not the case. We see the world through a filter of our own thoughts, experiences and beliefs. When we express an opinion, we are describing our own selves, and if anyone disagrees with our perception we feel an affront and immediately assume they are deluded. This applies to our own view of ageing too. The problem is our view of ageing describes how we see ourselves as older people, and this is likely to be a self-fulfilling prophecy, for anything else would mean accepting the humiliating idea that our perception was wrong. Selective perception has major implications for our health. Our perceptions of how long we have to live directly affect our physiology. Let us favour the Aha! moment more often. Opening our minds to other possibilities will enrich life; believing we will live long after the age of eighty in a state of mental and physical fitness will increase the probability this perception will come true.

The Problem of Generosity

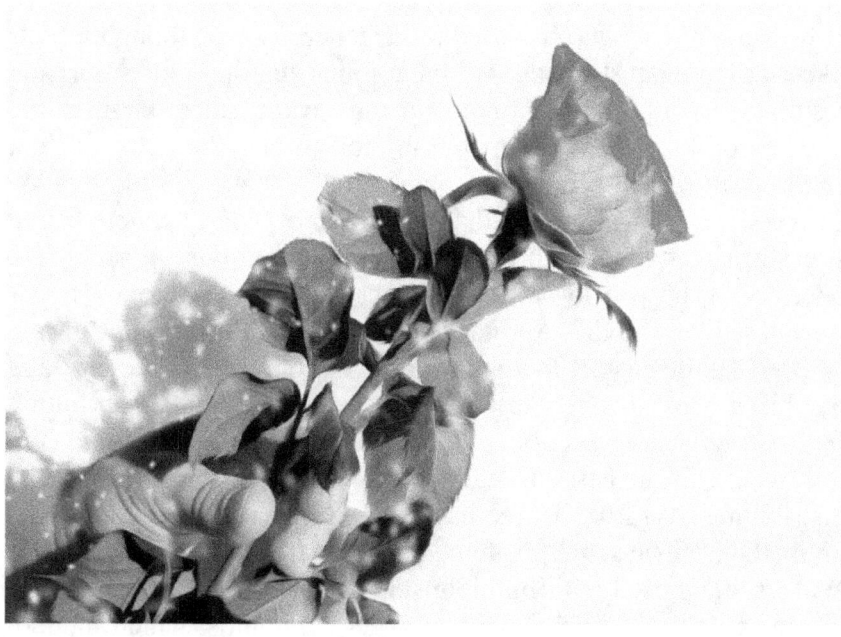

For those of us who find generosity challenging, being told we should be generous can trigger a host of feelings of resistance and guilt that leaves us feeling we are lacking, while not wishing to remedy the lack. Generosity can be difficult for those who had a less than ideal childhood. Watching one's family members cut out grocery coupons and worry about money, discuss prices and wring their hands over taxes and bills makes a strong imprint on a child and informs his or her attitude to money later on. Furthermore we are constantly told we live in a world of shrinking resources, that only the few will make it to the top, and that less and less will be available as time goes by. Society also adjusts to any increase in abundance by decreasing what is on offer – thus a single salary was enough for a family to live on in the nineteen seventies, but today the same standard of living requires two salaries. This is the law of diminishing returns. Set against such a social cue, it is extremely difficult for many of us to give anything away for free, or to believe that an act of generosity will yield more abundance in the long run.

However, anyone who has tried to be generous even though it feels like battling against a gale will have found that it yields surprising results. It is, for example, good for our health, since it causes the release of oxytocin – important for social bonding – and endorphins, which reduce the perception of pain. A study at the University of Buffalo found that in a group of elderly people facing stressful situations (death of a family member, financial problems, burglary...) those who had helped others during the previous year were less likely to die. Andy Mackie, dubbed the Harmonica Man, stopped taking his 15 medicines after his ninth heart surgery and put his money towards teaching students music and distributing free harmonicas to schoolchildren. Although his doctors told him this would mean certain death, he lived almost ten more years, distributing over 20,000 free harmonicas with the money he saved on medicine. The same phenomenon affected South African Camie Walker, diagnosed with multiple sclerosis. Advised by a medicine woman to give 29 gifts in 29 days, her symptoms, which modern medicine could not cure, began to disappear. Further studies have shown that giving to a worthy cause activates the same brain regions as food, sex and earning a bonus for oneself. Giving activates the relaxation response and subsequently the body's natural repair mechanisms.

It sometimes helps to take a banknote and ask ourselves what it really is. The note is composed of paper, with some fibre. Its lifespan is about two years. Its intrinsic value is minimal – it simply represents something. If it represents what we have in the bank, what then is this? Our bank accounts are now merely virtual. They exist in cyberspace, and appear in the form of a series of numbers on a screen. What then is this money stuff? Is it not simply a form of energy, an agreement as to how much of ourselves we have put out there? A value based on a social agreement, on other people's perceptions? Money is created by a kind of a perpetual interaction between concrete things, our

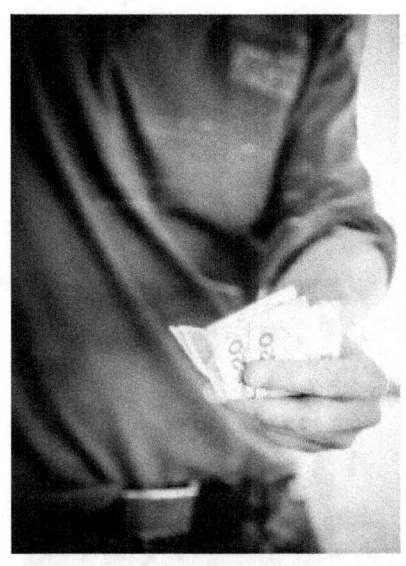

intangible desire for them and our abstract faith in what has value. Money is valuable because we want it, but we want it only because it can get us a desired product or service.

A shift of perspective is necessary to start the flow of events an act of generosity triggers, so for those of us who feel anxiety when we give to others, let us try with something small – volunteering to do a chore, or to buy a round of coffee, or food for someone, stop to give directions or stay on after hours to help someone in need. Then let us observe how we feel inside – gently does it, no need to force this. If this feels good, we can then progress to larger acts of generosity as an experiment. Let us also observe our attitude to the rich – do we see them as selfish money-grabbing exploiters, or as generous supporters of charities? If we were rich, how would we give?

Many spiritual movements – including Christianity which says it is in giving that we receive – claim that those who give freely always get more back than they give out. This may be simply to do with feeling less anxious about money, less afraid of large amounts or what might happen to us if we lose money. But it may be something deeper – a more universal truth about the collective consciousness and the flow of energy between members of the group. If we are all part of the same life force, then giving away may create a vacuum of energy which sucks energy back in. The more we give – of time, love, money – the more we will suck back into our space. It's worth a try. It is an expression of self-love, since we know we will benefit more from a generous act than from clinging to what we have.

The Overpopulation Argument

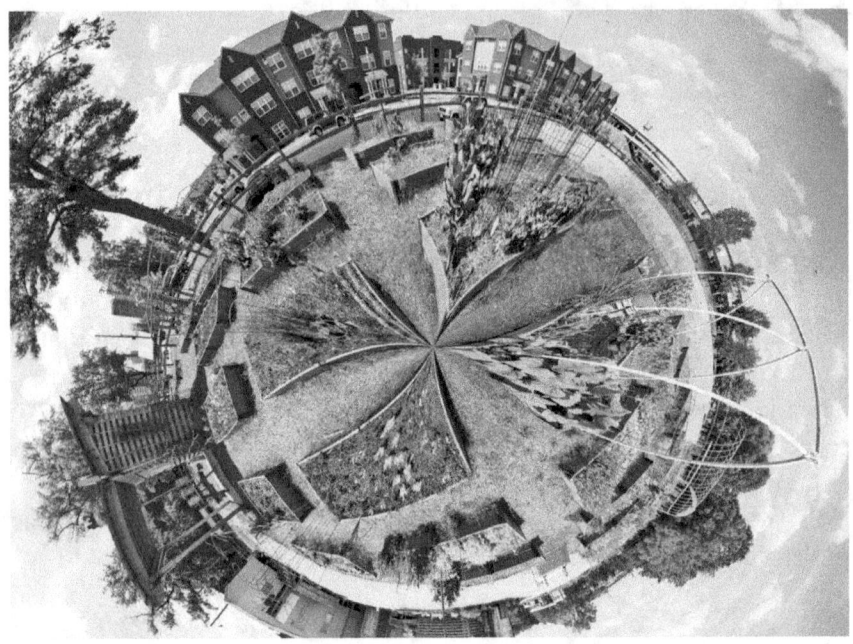

One of the major arguments against life extension is that our planet could not cope with a massive increase in the number of people, placing huge pressure on resources. However, much of the evidence to support this claim is quite easy to debunk. The World Health Organisation estimates that the world's population is going to double in the next fifty years. But this is based on current birth rates, and in the developed world these rates are already at an all-time low. The low number of children per woman (currently under 2 in the US and UK) may extend to poorer countries as planned parenthood becomes more widespread and education levels among women rise. The greatest impact on population as a result of life extension is going to be in countries that have low fertility rates anyway, so the population change would not be as great as one

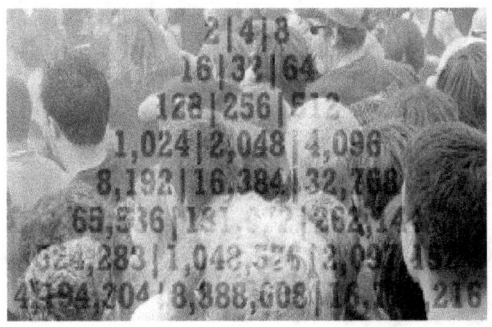 might fear. The same fears of the dangers of overpopulation were expressed in the 1970s because of a population boom; the catastrophe never materialised however because the predictions failed to factor in technological and agricultural progress. In fact, although there are six times as many people on the planet now than there were in 1800, we have better quality of life than ever before.

Social structures have been developed to deal with a lifespan where people retire at 65 and die at 80. As lifespan lengthens society will evolve with it, so that we may become used to not just two or three, but perhaps four or five generations around the table at a family reunion. Career structures would change, as people might choose to have a number of professions in their lifetime rather than one – this is already happening. Pension funds would make more long-term investments as people begin to draw a pension later in life, or continue to work and draw a reduced pension.

The wisdom and experience of having more older individuals alive, who are also likely to be healthier due to cutting edge research into what causes the body to age, would benefit the work place, politics, education and psychology. Younger people would no longer feel under such pressure to juggle family and work, since there would be no sudden vertical drop in income level at 65. Living longer would mean people would be more keen to protect the environment since they would have to live in it longer, perhaps two centuries. Medical costs would plummet as the battle against age-related disease is won, since most governments spend the largest proportion of their health expenditure on cancer, strokes and heart disease.

Fears of overpopulation are not a sufficiently strong argument to reject life extension. It is possible that within 30 years science will have identified the major longevity genes and will have sound proof of what lifestyle patterns prolong life. Some experts calculate that many people alive today will be still alive 150 years from now. Will we be among them?

We're Doomed!
(Pessimism as a life philosophy)

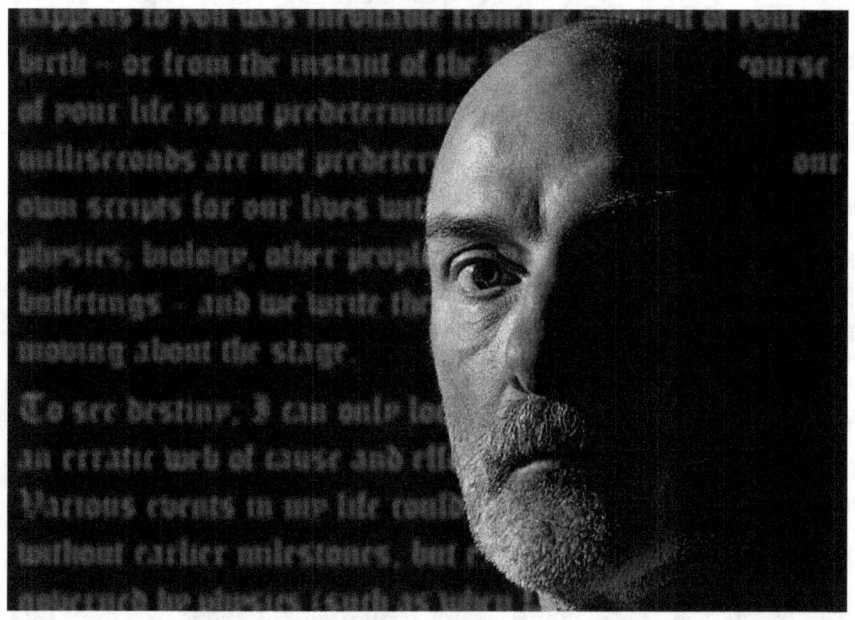

Do we need pessimists?

A positive thinking revolution has gripped the world in the wake of successes such as *The Secret*. Criticism of this revolution hinges on the idea that fantasising about our dreams coming true can distract us from taking the practical steps towards achieving them. Writing down the obstacles in our way, it is claimed, is a far more realistic approach to attaining a goal.

Psychology differentiates between two main types of pessimist. The first is the philosophical pessimist. This worldview challenges the idea advanced by the German philosopher Hegel of a world spirit of progress, with which the entire human race marches

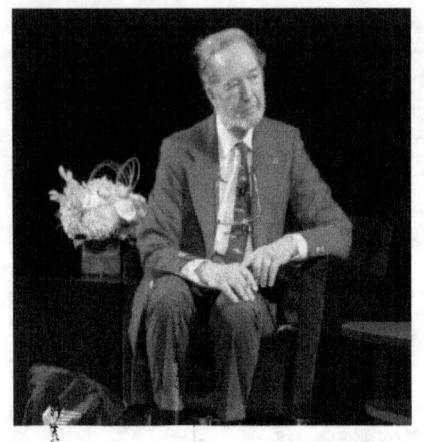

forward towards more freedom and rationality. It believes life has no intrinsic value, and that anything we do is ultimately meaningless. Able to contemplate the past and the future, humans cannot but be aware of the impermanent nature of life and our helplessness in the face of our ultimate demise. Far from advancing from one generation to the next, philosophical pessimists believe that even if technology brings about positive change, human beings cannot evolve and may even be regressing, becoming more corrupt as society becomes more complex. The human condition is therefore absurd.

The second form is depressive pessimism, which is more a state of mind brought about by a certain way of thinking. Therapists view this as unrealistic, and treatment involves bringing awareness of a patient's biased view of the world. The theory is that depressive pessimists feel more comfortable believing in the worst possible outcome, since this enables them to manage anxiety and avoid disappointment. They are more likely to blame themselves when something doesn't go well, since their worldview is often coloured by a lack of confidence, which can be the first step in a spiral of depression. However, sometimes depressive pessimists are successful in life if they use their gloomy outlook to minimise risk, in business for example, since they may apply their pessimism to planning carefully in order to survive and calculate the way to attain the best possible outcome. Some may be able to reduce or eliminate anxiety to the point where they can be better described as strategic, rather than depressive pessimists.

But surely being permanently in a pessimistic frame of mind cannot be the best way to manage life overall. Pessimism is linked to joylessness and misanthropy, and pessimists spread an atmosphere of gloom that may prevent others from taking positive action, even if they themselves are actually doing well. Positive feedback about how we are doing always spurs us on to higher ground, and no dog-in-the-manger pessimist is going to offer encouragement and thanks for a job well done, since pessimism has at its heart a belief that whatever we do, life is pointless. On the other hand, excessive optimism can become toxic if it ignores the challenges to come, and the fall when the hoped-for outcome doesn't materialise can be painful, even shocking. The pessimist in a group can serve as a security fence to remind us that unplanned outcomes should be factored in.

The best way of giving ourselves the correct dose of optimistic realism is to do a body scan and see what feels good to us, since we are all different. Inertia and defeatism help no one. Pessimism may provide a necessary dose of vigilance. The question is, how do we regard someone who lived their entire life as a pessimist and then died? Did they live life well?

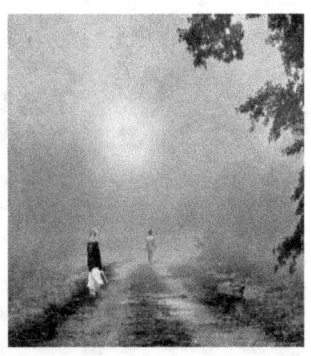

The Inner Monologue

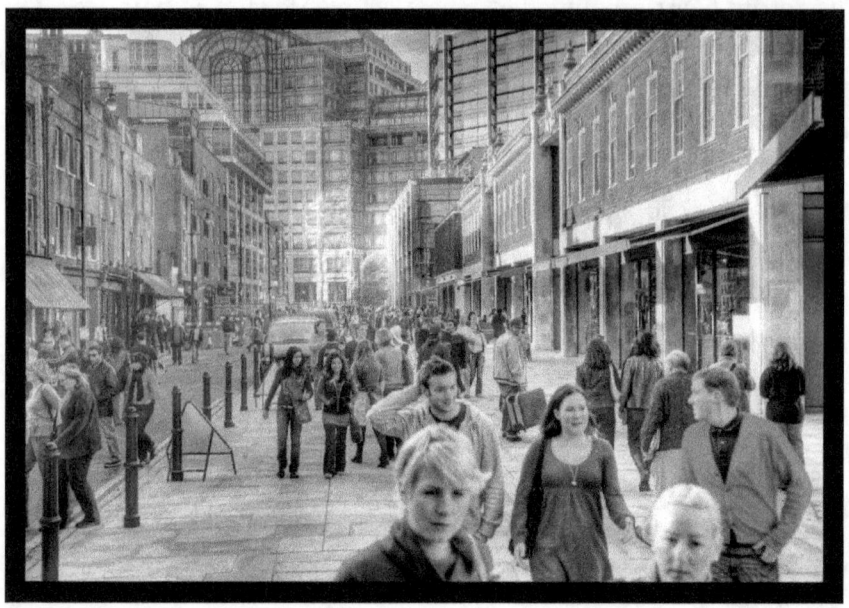

What do you say to yourself when no one is around? Take a crowded street. Every one of the individuals will be experiencing an inner or outer monologue. We are all part of the hive and the astonishing density of human thought emitted by our planet on a daily basis makes up the collective consciousness. It is constant, mainly unstoppable and can sometimes prevent us from falling asleep at night. Some of the people on that street will be running through the filing cabinet of their minds – speech rehearsal, appointment planning, phone call scheduling etc. Others will be reviewing recent events, the classic "post-mortem" of a confrontation, a successful conversation or a piece of work completed. Common thoughts are feeling we are an imposter at work ("Well, I fooled them all yet again. One day they're going to find me out."), fear we will lose love ("He's going off me. It's my thighs."), or steeling ourselves against life ("Don't give up. You

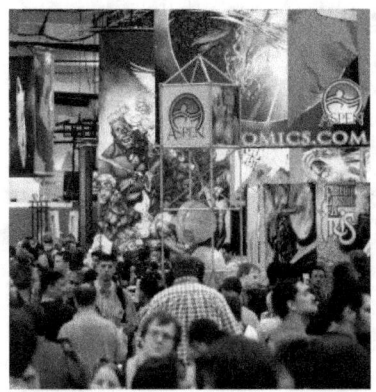

can do it. So-and-so believes in me."). Still other pedestrians will be analysing how their lives are going ("I have a shoulder pain. It's cancer, I know it," or "I'm going to get home and there'll be another lawyer's bill waiting," or "I worked well today. And the boss noticed.") This form of analysis has little to do with outside events and everything to do with our default setting of how we see the world. Most of the people will be flitting in a seemingly random way from one form of inner monologue to the next.

Stream of consciousness is slightly different; it tends to be less ordered than interior monologue. In literature, stream of consciousness has little or no punctuation, and in the mind this may take the form of flashes of concepts, pictures, or ideas without verbalisation or sentence construction.

A conversation with oneself is one of the few mental activities humans can actively observe, the other tasks of the brain being largely unconscious or automatic. The inner monologue depicts activity in the prefrontal cortex which is associated with logic and reason. In those suffering from schizophrenia, the internal dialogue will depict active areas all over the brain, illustrating the person's inability to distinguish between their own thoughts and the reality outside.

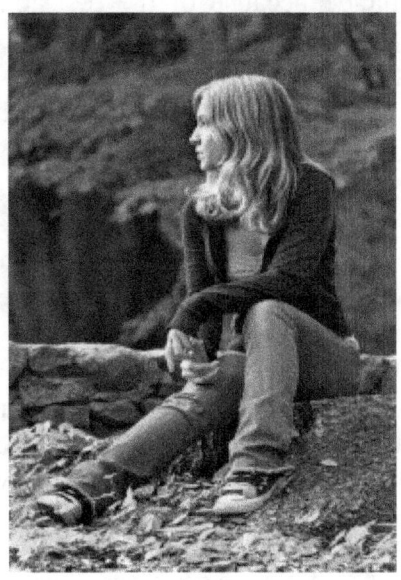

If we are serious about staying ageless and living fulfilled lives it is important to begin to monitor this inner monologue. The stories we tell ourselves affect our mood, and vice versa. Our perception is rarely completely objective, and those of a pessimistic, fatalistic disposition are more likely to have paranoid or defeatist thoughts. These emotional states can have an enormous impact on how we proceed along the arrow of time. Successful people will see a negative event as a springboard for a learning experience or for a future success. Defeatist individuals will see setbacks as confirmation of their own lack of worth, or their constant stream of bad luck, or of the pointlessness of trying. Let us be under no illusions: the inner monologue is independent of actual events. The same events will trigger a completely different inner monologue in different individuals. Moreover the stories we tell ourselves are coloured by our culture and our family environment. This is why it is important to protect ourselves against fundamentalist pessimists in our entourage.

Two examples spring to mind : recently Amnesty International profiled the case of Amina Filali, a 16 year old who committed suicide because of the decision of a judge to marry her to her rapist, a common "solution" to rape cases in Morocco. Let us imagine her inner monologue as she prepared to end her life. How could she have changed it? Another example is that of Lily. She was belittled in her childhood and overshadowed by her successful sister. When her true love, the one who could have taken her into adulthood with him, preferred another girl, her world collapsed, she contracted cancer of the thyroid, increased the drinking she had innocently copied from her father and went into rapid decline. She then spent the next 20-30 years thinking she was worthless and a burden to everybody. In fact she was far from that, being a very artistic and humane woman, and earnt her welfare payments by manning after-school homework classes for underprivileged children, teaching art classes as well as being an anonymous phone counsellor. But changing her inner monologue could have changed her life.

Some of us may have heard of the 1950s B-movie, *The Attack of the 50 Foot Woman*. When it comes to our thoughts, we must protect ourselves against the attack of the 50 foot inner monologue. Vigilance is everything. Let us clean up our mind today, and prepare for change.

Are you receiving me?

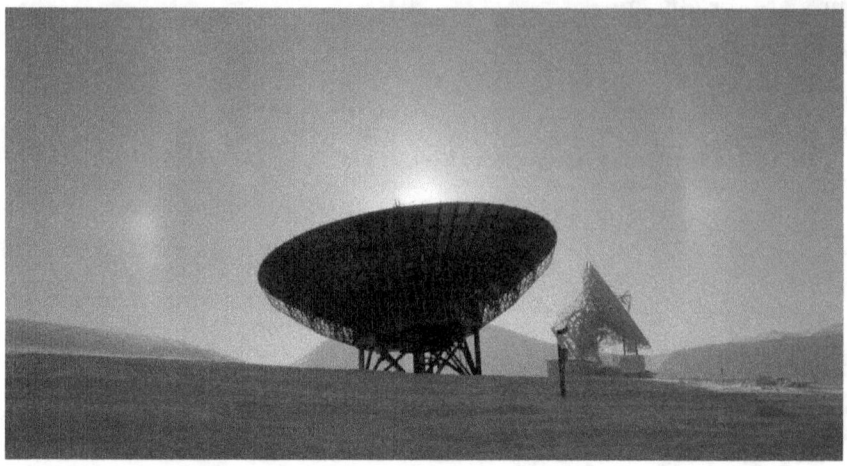

Receptors are message receivers located on the surfaces of cells, which initiate a sequence of changes in our bodies : for example, changes in the use of energy, tissue growth or the perception of pleasure and pain. These receptors receive hormones and neurotransmitters, which lock onto the receptors and trigger the event. When there is an excess of a certain hormone, first receptor resistance occurs and then the number of receptors decreases. There is some evidence that obesity is in part caused by a deficit in dopamine receptors. This leads the obese to overeat to achieve the level of satiety that normal individuals reach with less food. Bingeing raises the level of dopamine even higher, which leads to resistance and a 'down-regulation' of dopamine receptors, only worsening the craving problem. Genes may cause the initial problem and poor diet exacerbates it. Low levels of dopamine receptors are also found in alcoholics and drug addicts. Cocaine, or heroine, bind to the receptor, causing dopamine to accumulate since it no longer can get in.

While dopamine receptors are located largely in the brain, serotonin receptors are to be found all over the body – 80% are in other organs. Depression has been linked to low dopamine and serotonin receptor levels. Antidepressants can therefore make things worse in the long run since they temporarily raise the amount of serotonin in the body but this saturation decreases the number of serotonin receptors. In all these cases – depression, obesity and addiction – receptors react to excessive levels of hormone by becoming less sensitive to them. The good news is we can also increase the number of receptors - for serotonin, dopamine and in the case of diabetes for insulin - since diabetes is caused by low levels of insulin receptors. Intense exercise, particularly on an empty stomach, resensitises receptors, and increases their number. In this way satiety from food and pleasure from life is more easily achieved. Fasting works in the same way. A decline in dopamine receptors is associated with ageing, but once again here is evidence a symptom of ageing can be reversed.

If we have enough dopamine receptors life becomes more than merely bearable. It is not just worth living, it becomes a source of fascination and adventure. Dopamine receptors enable us to max out on pleasure. Biology is not destiny and the decline associated with ageing is not inevitable. There is no quick fix, but a sustained exercise programme and calorie restriction can work wonders.

Stoicism and the Art of Self-Denial

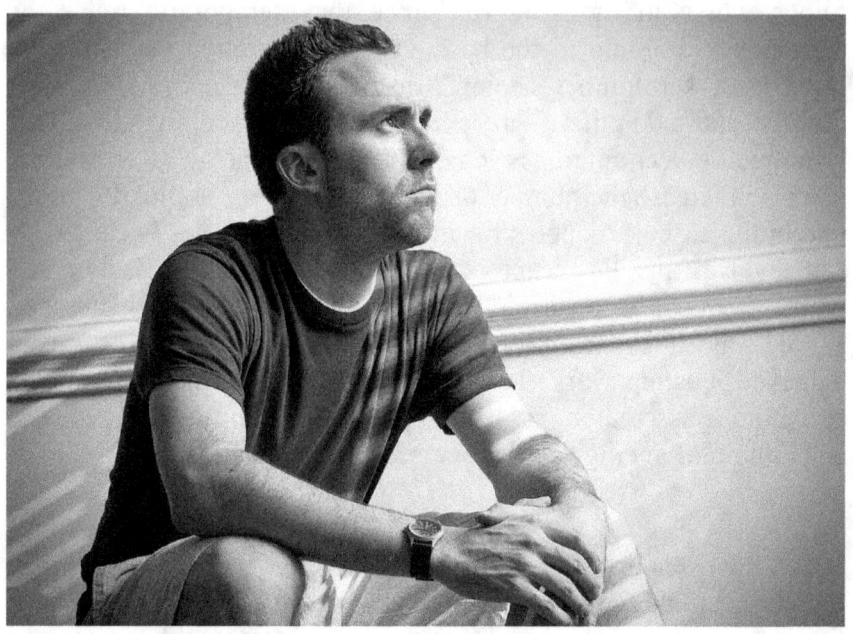

The Stoics believed that by controlling our minds we can control our world and ultimately our destiny – not unlike the law of attraction that has gained so many followers today. For the 3rd century BC Stoics, negative emotions were the result of wrong thinking. Distress was the result of being of the opinion that something is bad and that the only possible response is feeling distressed. When we feel that the world has done us a disservice, it is not uncommon for our inner monologue to imagine explaining our distress to others : in this way we justify our sorrow and indignation to ourselves. Stoicism taught self-control and reason with the aim of being free from rage, jealousy and depression. Marcus Aurelius was a Roman emperor in the 2nd century and a follower of stoicism. In his meditations he says:

"Say to yourself in the early morning: I shall meet today ungrateful, violent, treacherous, envious, uncharitable men. All of these things have come upon them through ignorance of real good and ill... I can neither be harmed by any of them, for no man will involve me in wrong, nor can I be angry with my kinsman or hate him; for we have come into the world to work together..."

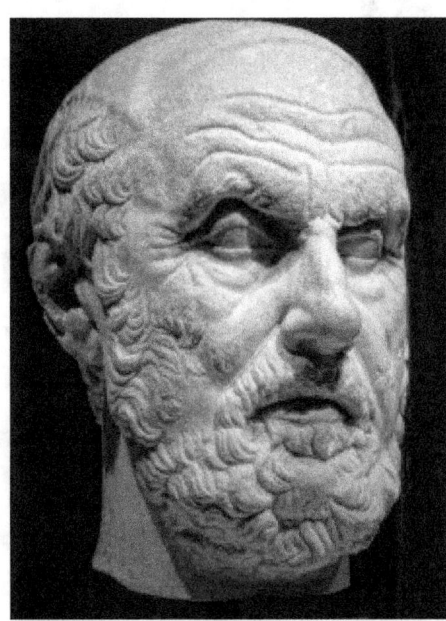

Clear-thinking and a philosophy of virtuous living is the basis for all philosophies and religions, but it is the Stoics' aversion to self-pity that makes stoicism timeless. Marcus Aurelius echoes Byron Katie's epiphany when she woke up from her years of depression in 1986 in advising : get rid of the thought *I am hurt*, and you get rid of the hurt itself. Attitude is therefore everything.

Stoicism is often maligned as being about emotional detachment and self-obsession, the stiff upper lip which engenders insensitivity to others. What is less known is that the Stoics advocated the cultivation of happiness and benevolence towards their fellow men. The real self-denial of a Stoic is denying oneself destructive thoughts and attitudes. They advocated enjoying pleasures without being dependent on them ("mastery of passion"), feeling joy in our relationships to others without the fear of loss and overcoming mistreatment by others through practical techniques, so that we may be sick yet happy, in disgrace and yet at peace. The Stoic Epictetus said, "Men are not disturbed by events, but by their opinion about events." Wallowing was a reflex they subjected to personal will. Exercising will power was, to them, like exercising a muscle – the more we use it the stronger it gets. Physical and mental self-control was the key to a successful life.

The principles of stoicism have been adapted to modern-day cognitive behavioural therapy, which treats patients with depression and trauma. History is full of individuals who applied these principles to overcome suffering – captured soldiers in times of war, people born with a disability, those facing famine or epidemics or natural disaster. If we have faced adversity in our lives, and bounced back, we are a modern-day stoic.

Adversity is nothing more than an opportunity for greatness. Overcoming stressful situations can actually promote health. Stoicism is not a dry, joyless antiquated ideology; it has much to offer for the foundations of a successful, long life.

Photo Credit: mharrsch via Compfight cc
Photo Credit: christopherdale via Compfight cc

The Slow Metabolism – Nature's Greatest Gift

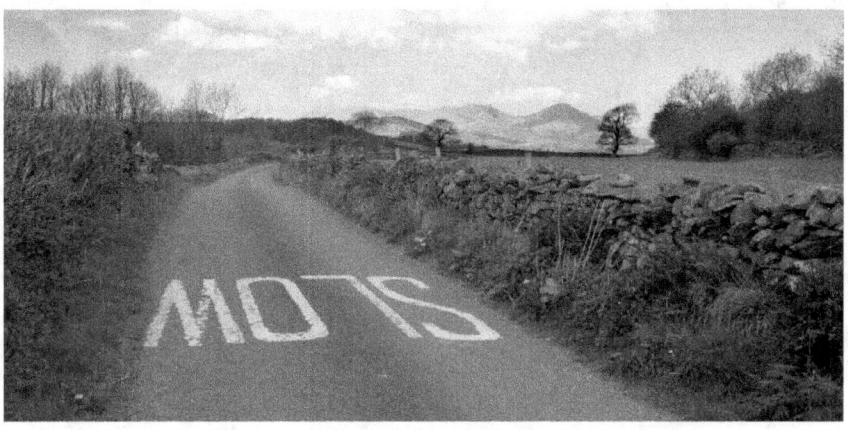

Something of a dilemma has emerged recently regarding metabolism in the healthy living community. Most people want to speed up their metabolism. Those of us who have always had a weight problem will no doubt remember watching skinny kids devouring biscuits and chocolate at break time at school, knowing that if we were to do the same we would be enormous, and subject to even more taunting. The medical community has always told us that it's not about metabolism, but about our food and beverage intake and our physical activity, but anyone with a weight problem knows this is simply not true. There clearly are people who eat much more than plump people and never gain weight, and there are people who run every day or hit the gym several times a week and still can't lose the beer gut. Some people just seem to have slim genes. But of course, if we diet, our body doesn't set about losing the fat as we want it to; instead something even worse happens – it starts stocking even more fat because it thinks it's in starvation mode, and when we come off the diet, we end up fatter than ever.

But now…things are changing. Is a fast metabolism really such great news, or are those of us heaving around a sluggish metabolism actually secretly blessed with the greatest gift nature could bestow?

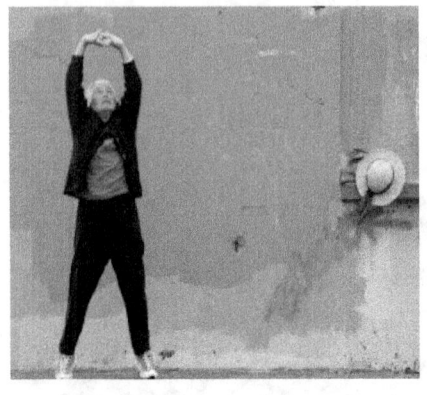

What happens when we burn food fast? Our body says, I need more, so we feed it regularly. Every time we eat toxins are produced. If we have a fast metabolism and have to refuel constantly, evidence is emerging it will wear out faster. In animals, daily energy expenditure is indeed inversely related to lifespan. By reducing calorie intake while continuing to meet the body's needs for nutrients, daily energy demands are reduced. Oxidative damage goes down (the by-product of metabolism). So the less we eat, the healthier we are. Those of us who have learnt to eat less so as not to gain weight, especially if we have been doing this from childhood, are in the running for a longer, healthier life.

So what of exercise, which causes our metabolism to work faster? How come exercise is also linked to longevity? The point here is the free radicals produced during exercise are quickly eliminated by the body, with the added bonus that the body produces antioxidant enzymes right afterwards, which means the body is better at protecting itself all day long.

Calorie restriction diets make us lose weight at first but – as all dieters know - over time, our body adjusts its metabolism to fit the lower calorie intake, and we stop losing weight. Contrary to what the yo-yo dieters have always thought, this is good! Keep calorie intake low *permanently* and avoid chronic illness and accelerated ageing.

So managed correctly, a slow metabolism is a fabulous gift. And those of us who were born with a fast one can adjust our

142

metabolism to slow down, so that life itself slows down, giving us more years in better health.

Obesity is to be avoided at all costs; instead let us use nature's gift of a slow metabolism to train our body to function with less. Exercise-induced rises in energy expenditure are still associated with increased, not decreased, longevity. Although exercise increases free radical production in the short-term, the body adapts to these free radicals. When it does, it becomes even better at protecting itself against their damaging effects by producing more cell-protective antioxidant enzymes.

Photo Credit: hey mr glen via Compfight cc

Will bullies also live forever?

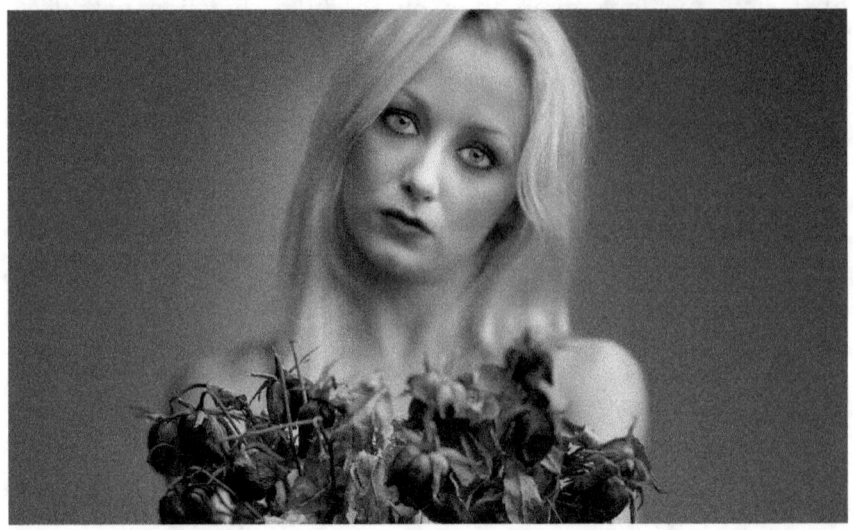

There is a taboo subject surrounding the death of certain people we know. It is the feeling of relief.

When they pass away, acquaintances and relatives who have in some way blighted our lives, either knowingly through abuse, or unconsciously through placing their own expectations upon us, can free us to explore many new possibilities. Feeling relief at the death of a parent whose disapproval or mockery we feared is an extremely common phenomenon, but to express it seems callous, and our feelings are often mixed, so we keep them to ourselves. Sabine, a woman in her early sixties from Austria says, "My father was a tyrant. He terrorised my mother who died of a heart attack in her fifties, and beat my brothers. I was his golden girl, but he ruined my youth by spoiling our family life. We were constantly walking on eggshells. I moved to another country as soon as I was able, but his disapproval of the fact I had a child out of wedlock cast a shadow over my joy at being a mother. When he died I felt finally free."

How can we advocate living past 100, even to 150 as Sonia Arrison suggests will soon be possible in her book *100+*, when this might mean never being free of our parents, or of that 'friend' whom we find so difficult when she phones up, or of the boss who made us feel so small and whom we still occasionally see in town?

The question becomes even more pertinent when we examine the case of brutal dictators. However, this is not such a clear-cut problem, as Sonia Arrison argues: "In fact the longer a dictator lives the more likely it is he will create enemies and increase his vulnerability to being ousted and brought to justice."

Indeed, this is what happened with the Nazis and what would have happened to General Pinochet. The recent Jimmy Saville case in the UK is also a good example. The victims of this pedophile never got justice since he died before his actions came to the attention of the press and the police. He could not even be stripped of his knighthood since individuals cease to hold the honour after death.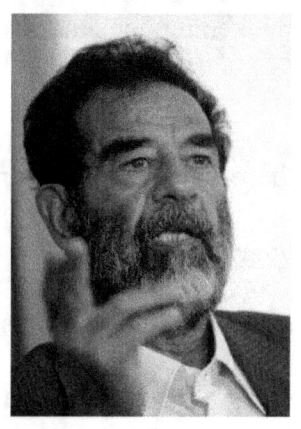

But what of the little dictators in the private sphere that blight the lives of people no one ever hears about? Those who may not commit actual crimes but whose bullying tactics for example, or emotional abuse keep their victims from happiness? We are talking of parents who continue a habit acquired in a child's early years of using them as a scapegoat for the family's problems – a trait common in narcissistic parents. We are talking about fathers who compete professionally with their sons, or sisters who adopt a sneering attitude to their younger siblings. We are talking also about neighbours-from-hell, CEOs with psychopathic traits and religious leaders with an iron grip on their followers. Death therefore brings freedom in dysfunctional families, and a new

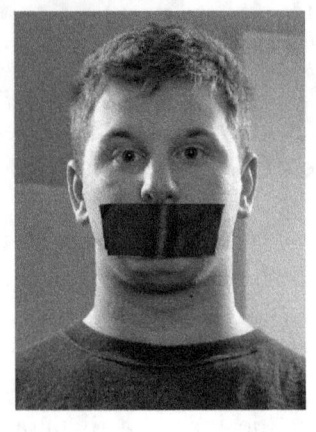

beginning in many social situations, so how can we square this with the drive to increase lifespan?

Life extension research more often than not focuses on genes and organ replacement, but it is our conviction that there is a spiritual dimension to living longer that is as important and probably more so. Stress avoidance and a positive attitude are part of this, but we would go further, and suggest belief that our health and vitality lies in our hands is an important factor in longevity. It depends on a mindful journey lasting a lifetime consisting in exorcising inner demons – negative emotions, trauma, life-weakening tendencies such as self-doubt, unworthiness, anxiety etc. but also traits that harm others such as rage, violence, jealousy and bullying. Overcoming the mental trauma caused by these states of mind and unlearning these unhelpful thought patterns is the way to avoid the stress that causes DNA damage. A longer life offers more possibility for reconciliation and mutual understanding, but this is clearly never going to happen with some people. It is our belief the conquest of the lower self is the key to long life, and those individuals who have failed to master their minds and emotions but who have nonetheless facilitated our spiritual growth are unlikely to be on that path, and are therefore not candidates for unusually lengthy lives.

Bullies are necessary. They make us appreciate their opposite, they throw love, tolerance and empathy into a brighter focus; they help us develop wisdom and fortitude. However, they are unlikely to be in our lives forever.

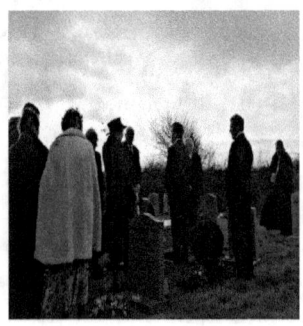

__The Inner Cavern__

A meditation

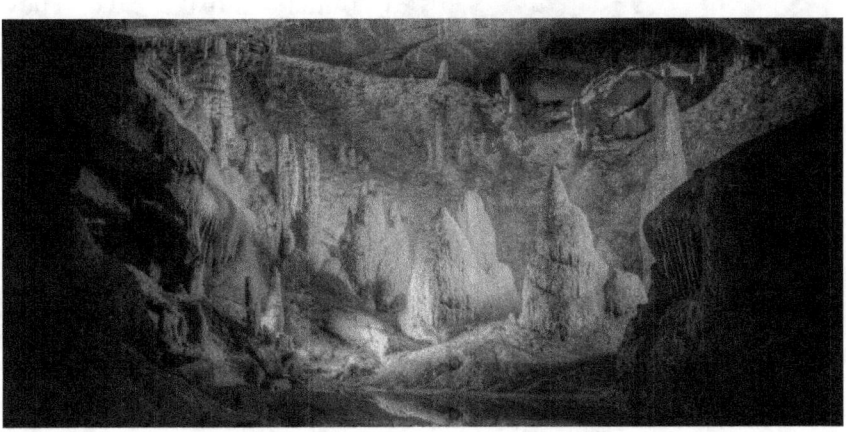

We are standing at the entrance to a cave. The bright sunlight behinds us slowly fades as we walk into the darkness and our eyes adjust to the light. Before us lies a subterranean lake, and at the shore, a boat bathed in light. We get in, and the boat lights our way as we travel across the lake in a grotto of breathtaking beauty. The glistening white rocks around us display cathedral organs of smooth stone, and there is the sound of slowly dripping water. Huge icicles hang down from the ceiling, and we arrive at the

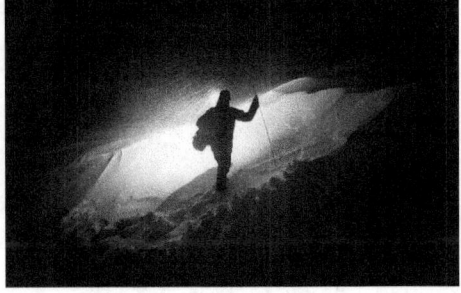

opposite shore, where we get out and contemplate a vast array of weird formations, a magic fairyland of glowing stalagmites rising up from the floor. Some of them seem to have had their tips chipped off.

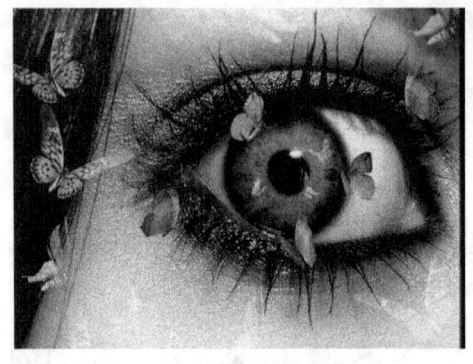

Suddenly we hear a soft hum, and a myriad of phosphorescent butterflies – purple, green, blue, whatever we choose – flutters into the cave. They seem to be attracted to the damaged formations in this surreal forest. Closer observation reveals they are depositing a resinous nectar on the ends, thick and dripping like treacle. Slowly the missing ends reform, the nectar solidifies and they are restored. The morphic field template that our bodies never lose recreates the original state of our damaged DNA; we have returned to our set point. Our set point is perfect health and youthful perfection. The butterflies are acting in accordance with commands from our consciousness. This is the mind-body connection which performs reverse engineering on damaged telomeres.

Satisfied that the wounds inflicted by accidents, past sickness, insults, abuse and trauma have been healed, we chant the mantra :

Peaceful ocean within me, be restored.
Om Nava Shivaya

(Meaning : "I bow to Shiva." Shiva is the inner Self. It is the name given to consciousness that dwells in everything. Shiva is the name of your true identity - yourself.)

This seals the repair work.

We then take the boat back across the lake, and go out into the sunlight, and continue our lives.

Pointlessness

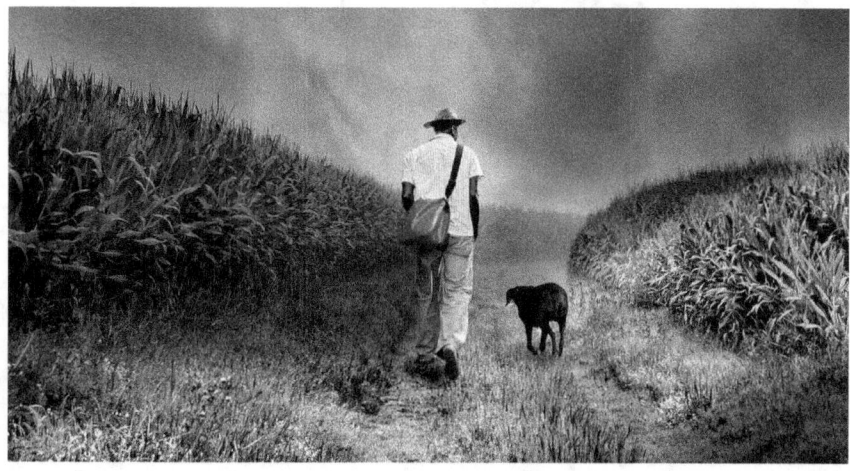

Life, looked at from a purely biological standpoint, is pointless. We are born, we reproduce, we die. Sometimes we don't even reproduce. So what is the point of extending life? If we're not into suicide, isn't the best thing to let old age have its way and get all that over with so we can go back to the far less taxing business of oblivion?

Of course, for those who believe there is life after death, the whole point of life is a learning, consciousness-expanding exercise. But atheists would say spirituality is the obvious knee-jerk response of all those billions of human beings who cannot cope with pointlessness. Futility is a concept that encompasses lack of importance, absence of purpose and being of no practical use. The Latin root means leaking away. Perhaps Nature went too far in giving us self-awareness. She should have stopped developing our brains at the level of cows, or fish. Then we'd be blissfully happy when alive and blissfully unaware of the concept of futility. Our lives would be sufficient unto themselves.

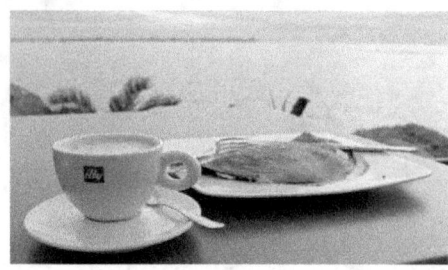 Feelings of pointlessness affect everyone from time to time, and some people feel it regularly, and are diagnosed with depression. Stress can lead to feeling fed up with life, since we are overwhelmed with things that need doing and seem to have no time to live ourselves. Being on the work treadmill, working as fast as we can just to pay the electricity and food bill, is the most common reason for a sense of pointlessness, combined with struggles in our personal relationships. When life stops being good it is time to stop and think.

Our small lives may have stopped being enjoyable, but the universe is so full of wondrous possibilities, this does not mean we cannot let some of that wonder in.

Is the life of a sparrow pointless? It is worth something simply because the sparrow is what it is.

Is the life of a bluebell pointless? Of course not, since without beauty the universe would be dark, and that *would* be pointless.

Are momentary feelings of happiness pointless? No they are not; they are worth living simply because they exist.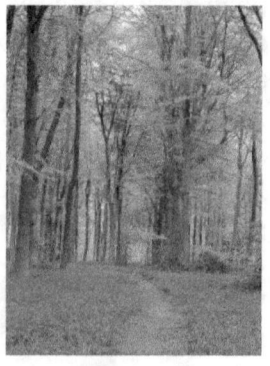

Why is there something rather than nothing? Because empty space would be pointless. Trying to find a point to life is akin to living constantly projecting towards the future, but life is worth living because of what we experience in the present. If that present is unpleasant, we must move ourselves gently to something else. One foot put gently in front of the other, as in a Tai Chi lesson where we must only follow the teacher's movements without any emotional or mental input, a slow and gentle walk towards a theatre, a park…changing our environment will change the lie in our mind that it is all pointless.

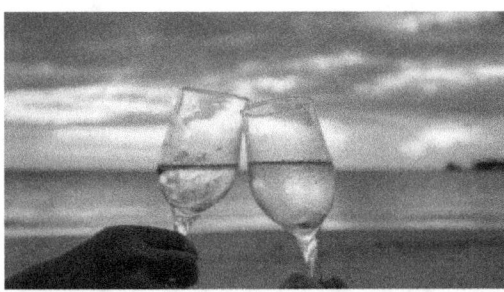 "I felt so down, so depressed at the end of my working day," said Donna, a single mother, "that I just wanted to throw myself off the railway bridge. I was working so much just to pay the bills for my children's education that I didn't have time to have any fun. I couldn't go on holiday without my children because I had no childcare, and yet desperately needed some down time without them to remember who I was. I was fed up of working outside and inside the home serving everyone else. What about me, what happened to *my* life, I wailed inside? That day I had signed up for a wine-tasting evening after work in an attempt to get myself to do other things. I did not want to go. I was too tired, too depressed and didn't want to see other people. But I made myself, and to help put one foot in front of the other I bought myself some chocolate; it helped, lifting my mood just enough to get me to the wine bar.

When I got there, I saw everyone else had come alone too. I began to talk to some of them, and forgot my dark thoughts. The wine expert was fascinating, and we all had a good giggle about how much wine we were putting away. I was astonished when I got home how my mood had changed. To think earlier on I had been contemplating suicide."

One act – deciding to go to the wine-tasting – changed Donna's perception. Life was worth living for the experience of tasting French wine with a group of friendly strangers. And therein lies the truth.

Photo Credit: gacabo via Compfight cc
Photo Credit: Aimanness Photography via Compfight cc
Photo Credit: h.koppdelaney via Compfight cc

__Watch Your Back__

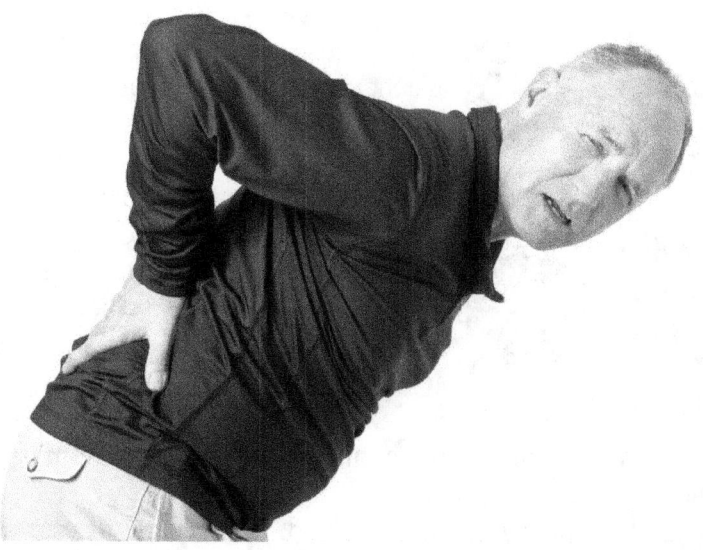

Back pain is one of the most common complaints known to man. We have the same spinal anatomy as all vertebrates, but it evolved for scampering around on four legs, so why did we emerge as the only upright quadruped if the price is searing pain in the back? Probably so that we could use our hands, but for those of us with aches and pains there does seem to be a design flaw. Organs are supposed to hang down *from,* not on a spine, babies are supposed to be carried underneath not in front – which is why human women have reinforcements at the base of the spine so they can get knocked up without getting knocked down.

Bad posture is one of the causes of back pain so regular posture checks throughout the day are a good idea – avoiding slouching and placing the shoulders in a comfortable position. We must pay attention not to lift more than 25% of our body weight, and make sure our work station is arranged so the chair is at the right height and the computer screen not too far away. Buying the right mattress – firm for some, softer for others – is important, and a pillow between the knees at night will provide extra lower back support.

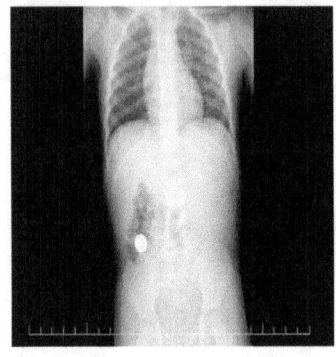

Other causes of pain include fractures, osteoarthritis, muscular problems, infections and illness. However, psychological factors are now emerging as a major factor in back pain. Depression, job dissatisfaction and passive coping strategies all contribute to chronic pain. Relieving emotional stress increases our ability to recover.

Apart from medication, active coping strategies include massage, physiotherapy and acupuncture, all of which have been demonstrated to promote mobility and pain relief. There is no reason to accept back pain as part of getting older.

It is important to note that one's attitude and life circumstances also have an effect on pain levels and duration. For example, people who are depressed, under stress or have a back injury are more likely to have their pain become chronic. Patients who are stress-free and have few complicating psychological factors are more likely to improve with appropriate treatment for their conditions.

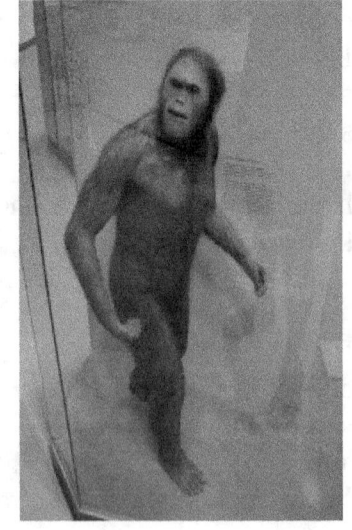

Finally, being fat was not part of the equation in the quadrupeds that stood up on their hind legs. Even today hunter gatherer communities are not known for complaining about back pain. It would be interesting to speculate what shape we would be if we had evolved to sit around on office chairs. In fact nature would never have allowed us to evolve as bipeds if extreme back pain were the trade-off. Back pain only becomes a problem in the context of modern life. Getting exercise (swimming is good because of the support from the water) and keeping the weight off as well as addressing stress immediately are the best ways to watch our backs.

The Woman God Forgot

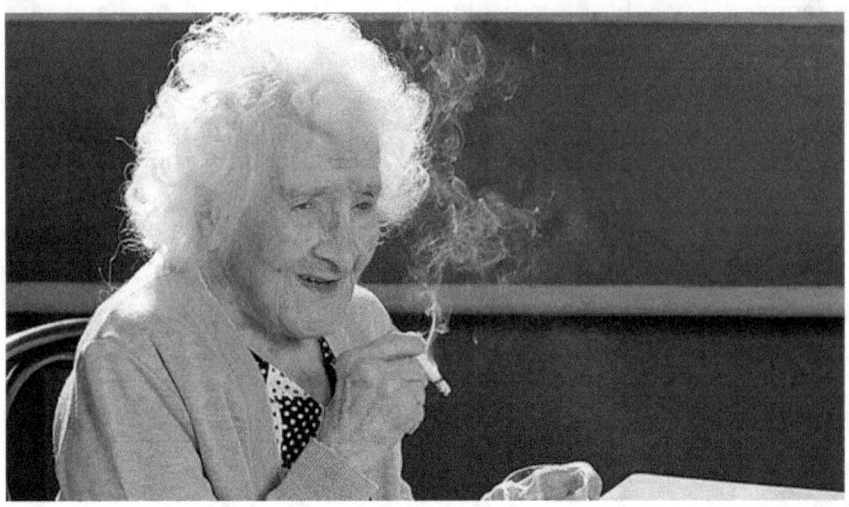

Jeanne Calment holds the world record for the longest confirmed lifespan. She lived in Arles, France, and claimed to have met Vincent van Gogh at the age of 13 when he came into her father's shop in 1888 to buy coloured pencils. She found him to be, "Dirty, badly dressed and disagreeable." She outlived her daughter and grandson by several decades. In 1965 she signed a deal to sell her apartment to lawyer André-François Raffray on a contingency contract. Then aged 47, he agreed to pay her 2,500 francs a month until she died. However, he died before she did, at 77 from cancer, and his widow was obliged to continue the payments – which ended up far exceeding the value of the apartment. Calment used to say to them that she was competing with Methuselah. She was 94 when man first walked on the moon, and lived on her own until the age of 110, when she moved into a nursing home having become blind and nearly deaf. Her mind was however still intact – until her death at the age of 122 she was sharp as a knife.

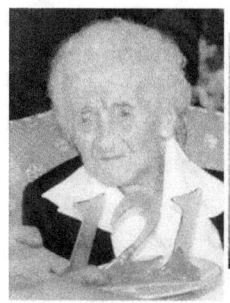 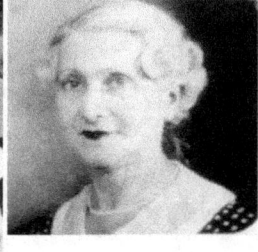

Jeanne at 121 years old   Jeanne at 60 years old

The assumption of the medics was that she benefited from extraordinary genes. Her father lived until six days shy of 93 and her brother François lived to the age of 97. Although genes probably played a part, there were also other aspects to her long life we can learn from. Her husband's wealth made it possible for her not to have to work; instead she lived a leisured lifestyle playing tennis, cycling, swimming, roller-skating, piano and going to the opera. Swimming in particular is a sport practised by many centenarians. At the age of 85 she took up fencing, proving that not sitting around waiting for death but developing new interests irrespective of age is a factor in life extension. The fact she continued to cycle until the age of 100 indicates regular exercise contributed to her longevity. It is also likely she suffered from very little stress. Not working is not an option for most of us, but it is nonetheless significant that she avoided all the diseases of later life while having a lot of fun. Managing stress through thought selection and intelligent use of music, massage/meditation and leisure is crucial to staying ageless.

She ascribed her long life to a diet rich in olive oil and garlic, which has been shown to help prevent arthritis, heart disease, hypertension and lung cancer among other things. She ate chocolate every day – today chocolate is lauded for its tremendous antioxidant potential. It lowers cholesterol, prevents cognitive decline and reduces the risk of cardiovascular problems. She also had a minor vice – a pêché mignon as the French say – port and a cigarette after her meal. Allowing oneself pleasurable things in moderation releases endorphins – or in lay terms, makes life worth living, proving the old adage that a little bit of what you fancy does you good. These days smokers can use e-cigarettes and

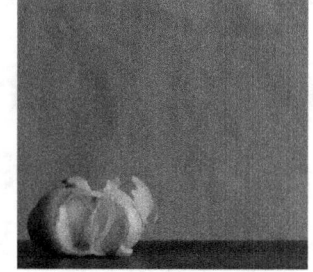

enjoy the pleasure of nicotine without the risks of tobacco. As she reached her 110th birthday she took to saying, "God has forgotten me". Her recipe for long life is telling – fun and laughter, or put another way, a positive outlook and developing the ability to avoiding casting oneself in the role of victim. When asked how she saw the future she replied with her famous sense of humour, "Short".

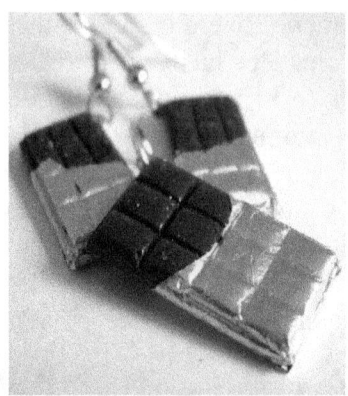

On her 122nd birthday on 21 February 1997 she decided not to make any more public appearances as her health had deteriorated. The French gerontologist Jean-Marie Robine said this "allowed her to die as the attention had kept her alive". He also said perhaps in a century everyone will live to 100.

Attitudes to ageing continue to change and medical research is unstoppable. Jeanne Calment died with a sound mind, but no one could claim she did not look her age. She was blind and almost deaf. Our goal is not to extend life to live it in feeble old age, but to live an active, healthy life to 100 and beyond.

After four and a half billion heart beats, her heart stopped on August 4th of the same year.

The Power of the Archetype

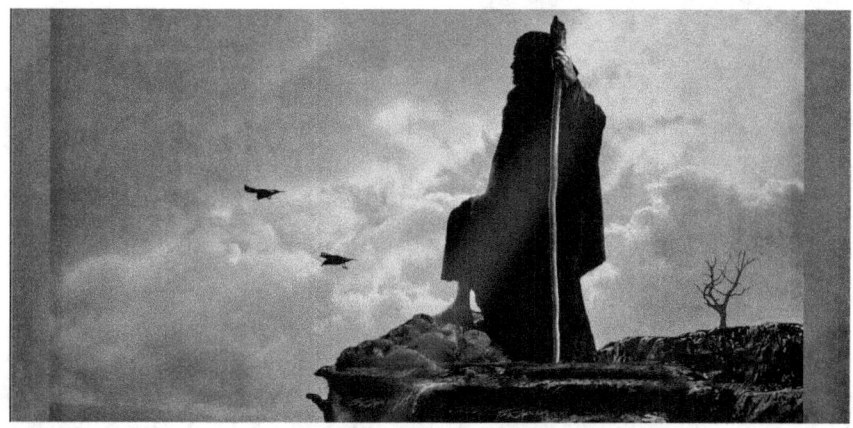

Archetypes are ideas or symbols that are present in everyone's mind. They symbolise patterns of behaviour and thought, and have been around ever since we became conscious beings on this earth. According to Plato, archetypal patterns are imprinted on the soul at the time of birth, but the psychoanalyst Carl Jung believed that they are separate energy forms that exist in the collective unconscious and which we tap into without realising. For Jung, archetypes form a bridge between science and religion, and between matter and spirit. They influence the way we think, feel, react to events and our value systems. Some mystics believe archetypes even influence the people we attract into our lives and the events we experience. They appear in mythology, literature and works of art. Archetypes are universal, and have both negative and positive faces.

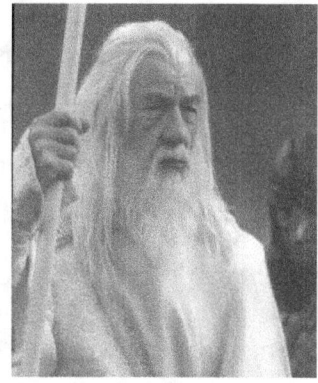

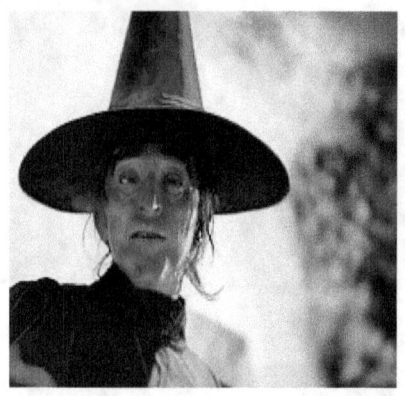

The archetype of the Elder is no exception. The male form can take the form of either the tyrant or the warrior. The tyrant is aggressive and not open to change. Blinded by his ego, his emotions are repressed. He is not interested in spirituality. The warrior however is both a father figure and a symbol of wisdom. He is successful, brave and capable of deep introspection. He is not afraid to confront his own demons. Which one are we headed for?

The female Elder archetype can take the form of the witch or the priestess. The witch is aware of the forces in this world, but uses them to justify her own ego. She is trapped in her own negative emotions, and prone to feelings of both victimhood and rage at the world for her fate. The priestess on the other hand is deeply intuitive, towards herself and other people's motives. She tries to understand others and gives advice only when solicited. Her humility leads her to question first herself before blaming others. She radiates wisdom, authority and unconditional love. Which one are we turning into?

Both the warrior and the priestess are aware of their connection to the collective unconscious. This awareness allows them to step outside received ideas and see societal trends for what they are. If we wish to stay ageless it is imperative that we question the assumptions our peers hold towards ageing. Most of us have been programmed from childhood to accept the archetype of the Elder as a weakling, with a declining mind and body, condemned to an

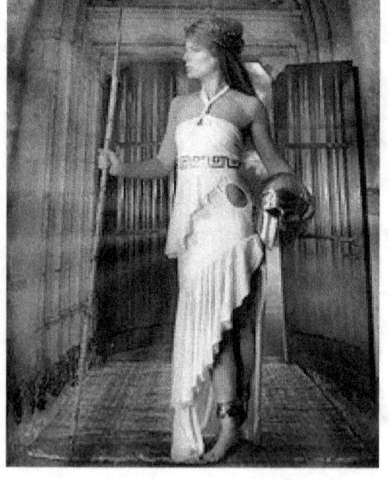

ever worsening quality of life, and death around 80. This is, however, an inherited idea; if there are examples of people who do not correspond to this archetype, we tend to dismiss them as exceptional. So-and-so is 'amazing for her age' – another might be 'still able to walk quite far unassisted' or 'capable of doing the Times crossword despite being over 90'. These subtle statements bear witness to programming that states being in good health after age 'X' (fill in whatever age you expect to go downhill) is generally not the rule, and that therefore we should not be disappointed if we do not "do all our own shopping", "manage the stairs" or "touch our toes without groaning" once past age X.

Archetypes are powerful tools that can tap into our subconscious for good or for bad. As vectors of the enormous influence of generations of our ancestors, they can linger at the back of our minds for decades and make an appearance in our lives after retirement, or manifest suddenly in our dreams at times of transition. They can aid us in moving onward and upward to more wisdom and achievement, or scupper any attempt we might have made to change for the better, sending us into a downward spiral of helplessness. Irrespective of our cultural background, we must remain aware of the power of the archetype, and ensure we master its influence, rather than allowing it to control us.

Expectations

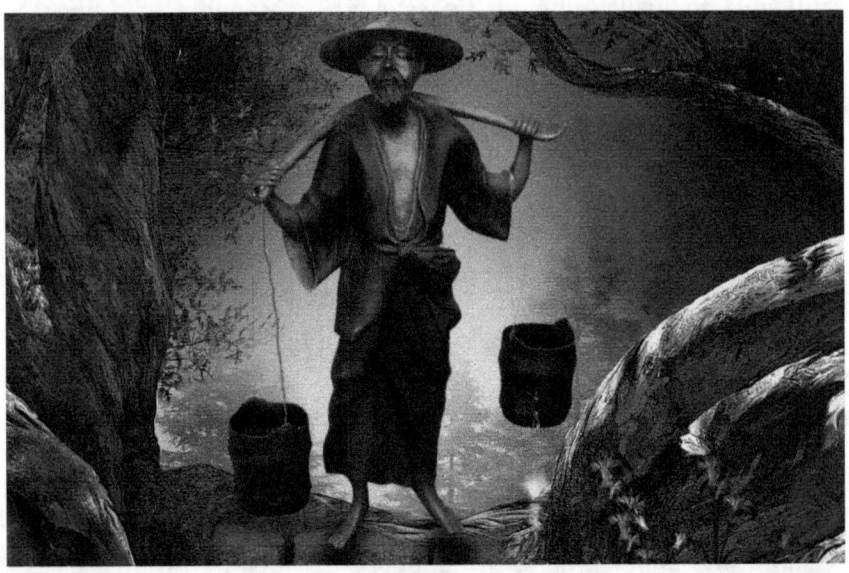

Near Yangshuo, southern China, there is a hill known as the Mountain of the Moon. It has 800 steps and in summer is an exhausting climb, necessitating several stops along the way. Water is sold by local people to the tourists on the way up. The vendors are mostly elderly people, many are tiny, thin women, and they haul dozens of bottles of heavy water up the steps countless times a day in the searing heat, dangling from a yoke. They not only keep pace with the young tourists they sell to (there are no elderly Westerners on the hike), but often overtake them. Their physiology is no different from ours; what is different is their expectations of their abilities. Expectations are a powerful feature of our psychology. Far from being mere thoughts about what might happen, sociologists such as Merton and Thomas have shown that expectations lead to behaviours and attitudes that cause the expectations to occur. Whether or not an expectation is based in reality has little or no effect on the outcome, since if someone has

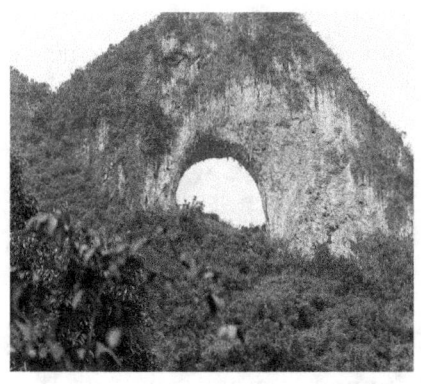

convinced themselves that something is true, or will occur, events will follow their conviction to their logical conclusion. The Thomas theorem states, "If men define situations as real, they are real in their consequences". According to Thomas, our behaviour is often determined by our perception of a situation we are in, and the meaning we ascribe to the situation. A young person with back ache will look for recent activity which may have led to the pain whereas the older person, even if they have engaged in the same activity, is more likely to ascribe the pain to advancing age. Once a person is convinced of something, they will take actions which are affected by their subjective perceptions – in the above case this could lead to a reduction in physical activity, which will then reduce fitness and lead to the corollary of expectations – the self-fulfilling prophecy.

There are many examples of self-fulfilling prophecies in society. A bank run is one, or in interpersonal relationships, a jealous woman who reacts strongly to her partner's contacts with other women so that eventually he feels so stifled he does indeed stray. A famous example includes a study where teachers were told arbitrarily that random students were "going to blossom". Oddly, those random students actually ended the year with significant improvements. In economics the life cycle theory shows that consumers pace their spending in accordance with how long they expect to live.

A self-fulfilling prophecy is based on "a false definition of the situation evoking a new behavior which makes the originally false conception come true" (Merton, 1948). To count, a belief must have consequences of a peculiar kind: consequences that make reality conform to the initial belief.

Thomas also stated that any definition of a situation will influence the present. After a series of such definitions, these perceptions gradually influence our mind-set and personality, so that our reality morphs into exactly what we had defined it to be. Is there any aspect of the way we regard our bodies which is causing a self-fulfilling prophecy?

In the new age movement, the power of expectations is known as the law of attraction, a belief that the universe will adjust itself to fit our expectations of the future. Though many have found this to be true, there is no scientific evidence as such. However, there is plenty of evidence for the placebo effect, where expectations that a medicine, however ineffective in reality, will work, leads to an enhancement of the immune system and the curing of disease.

It may seem that when we reach late "middle age", even if we have achieved our goals, the decline of the body must then be immediately addressed. It is as though we had a ledger in our minds indicating how long we have left. But what if the first 50 years were just a warm-up, and we could then return to the mental set point we had at 25, while maintaining all our knowledge and life experience…in other words, add on another full lifetime starting now? Would this change in attitude actually add those years to our life?

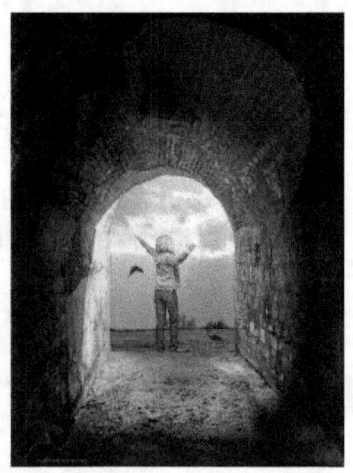

Fake it till you make it is not bad advice, although if we expect to stay in good physical and mental health up to our first century and to live well beyond there is no reason to believe this is fake. For some people this is already happening.

Photo Credit: violscraper via Compfight cc

Recommended reading :

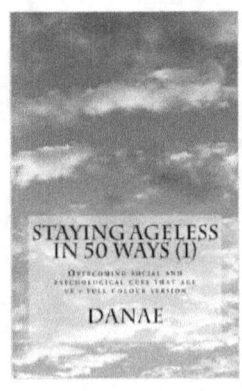

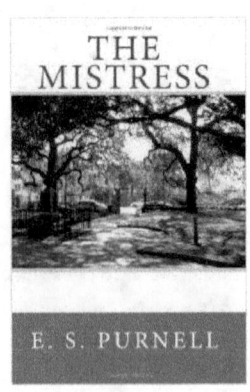